T0091623

Principles of Bone Regeneration

Jona J. Sela · Itai A. Bab
Editors

Principles of Bone Regeneration

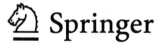 Springer

Editors
Jona J. Sela
Laboratory of Biomineralization
Institute of Dental Sciences
The Hebrew University Hadassah – Faculty
of Dental Medicine
Jerusalem, Israel

Itai A. Bab
Bone Laboratory
Institute of Dental Sciences
The Hebrew University of Jerusalem
Jerusalem, Israel

ISBN 978-1-4614-2058-3   e-ISBN 978-1-4614-2059-0
DOI 10.1007/978-1-4614-2059-0
Springer New York Dordrecht Heidelberg London

Library of Congress Control Number: 2012933362

Printed on acid-free paper

Springer is part of Springer Science+Business Media (www.springer.com)

Preface

Bone healing is the process whereby deficiencies and discontinuities in bone tissue are repaired by a regeneration process that rescues the biomechanical properties of the skeleton. Inevitably, this process involves an ultimate net gain in the amount of mineralized matrix at the affected sites. This gain may progress slowly, as in the case of the positive shift of bone remodeling balance induced in the osteoporotic skeleton by bone anabolic agents, or, as an outburst of bone formation and remodeling characteristic of the bone tissue reaction to traumatic insults. The importance of bone healing to medicine and biomedical research is illustrated by the number of publications on the different aspects of the subject, which exceeded 2,000 in 2011 alone.

Either form of bone healing is affected by a multitude of genetic, environmental, mechanical, cellular, and endocrine variables which eventually lead to changes in gene expression that enhance the guided action of osteoblasts (and chondroblasts) to lay down bone that restores, or even improves, the skeletal load bearing capacity and body motion. Needless to say, osteoclasts are also involved in shaping the healed tissue. Recent breakthroughs in understanding the regulatory aspects of bone formation and resorption, at the basic, translational, and clinical arenas, offer new modalities to induce, enhance, and guide repair processes in bone for the benefit of millions of patients with conditions such as osteoporosis, nonunion fractures, critical size defects, orthodontic tooth movement, periodontal bone loss, intraosseous implants, and deformed bones.

An immense number of approaches to treating these conditions are currently under basic, preclinical, and clinical investigations. They range from the development of sophisticated biomaterials for implant surgery, identification of neurotransmitters active in bone and other molecular drug targets, new drugs engineered by cutting edge pharmacological and molecular approaches, and advanced methods for tissue engineering and gene and cell therapies.

Because of the multidisciplinary nature of these efforts, this book addresses the modern aspects of bone healing, with a special attempt to enhance the convergence of the different experimental and clinical approaches designed for the study and treatment of bone healing in its diverse forms and under varying conditions. The information and ideas provided should have value not only for the experimental skeletal biologist and clinician treating bone conditions but also for a general interpretation of healing and regenerative processes in mammals.

Jerusalem, Israel   Jona J. Sela
                                                                            Itai A. Bab

About the Authors

Professor Jona J. Sela

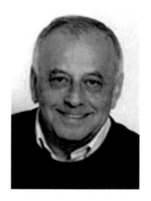

Born 1939, Jerusalem; D.M.D. 1966, Hebrew University

Appointments at the Hebrew University: Lecturer 1970; Senior Lecturer 1974; Associate Professor 1977; Professor 1981

Director, Division of Oral Pathology, 1989–2002

Chairman, Institute of Dental Sciences, 2004–2008

External Academic Positions

Honorary Research Fellow, Hard Tissue Unit, Department of Anatomy, University College London, UK, 1977

Visiting Scientist, Department of Human Genetics, UCL, UK, 1983

Lady Davis Visiting Professor, Department of Morphological Sciences, Bruce Rappaport Faculty of Medicine, Technion-Israel Institute of Technology, Haifa, Israel, 1986–1987

Guest Professor Medical Center Steglitz, Free University of Berlin, 1987

Chief-Superintendent, Head, Forensic Odontology, Israel Nat. Police 1987–1996; Chairman, Terminology Committees on Biological Sciences and Dental Medicine, The Hebrew Language Academy 1985–date

Visiting Professor UKBF, Free University of Berlin, Germany, 1996

Membership, Fellowship and Chairman

Chairman, Israel Society of Electron Microscopy, 1988–1993

NY Acad. of Sciences; Amer. Acad. of Oral Path.; Royal Micros. Soc.

Chairman, Jerusalem Branch, Israel Dental Assoc., 1970–1975. Founder, Chairman, Unit for First Aid, Magen David Adom, Jerusalem; 1972–1975

Secretary, 1978–1979, President, 1979–1980, Isr. Div. Int. Assoc. Dent. Res.

Isr. Soc. of Oral Pathology and Oral Medicine; Isr. Soc. of Anatomy

Int. Soc. of Forensic Odonto-Stomatology.; Eur. Soc. of Calcified Tiss.

Int. Assoc. of Oral Path.; Amer. Soc. Bone Min. Res.; Isr. Assoc Path.

President, Israel Soc. of Calcified Tissues, 1999–date. Fellow, the Royal Society of Medicine, London, UK

Research Interest and Projects

Gene-expression of bone cells around orthopedic implants. Automated image analysis supported by computerized quantitative morphometry for the study of observations obtained by electron and light microscopy in normal and pathological conditions. Development of novel computerized quantitative histomorphometric methodology to study oral and systemic pathological changes in cancer and wound healing.

Professor Itai A. Bab

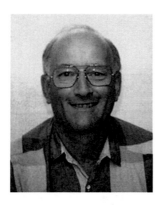

Born 1945, Rehovot, Israel. D.M.D. 1975, Hebrew University Jerusalem

Appointments at the Hebrew University: Lecturer 1979; Senior Lecturer 1982; Associate Professor 1986; Professor 1994

Research Interests and Projects

The bone laboratory is engaged in multidisciplinary research studying the mechanisms involved in skeletal remodeling, metabolic bone diseases, and the integration of endosseous implants. The laboratory studies the effects of different hormone and growth factor derived drugs on bone remodeling, bone mass, and healing of bone injuries. Recently, the laboratory has been engaged in the development of a new scientific field, neuropsychoosteology, which explores the bidirectional interaction between the brain and the skeleton. The methodological approaches employed in the laboratory encompass micro-computed tomography and histomorphometry, cellular and molecular biology, genetics, biochemistry and medicinal chemistry.

Endocannabinoids: Metabolites of Phospholipids as Modulators of Cell Function. Funding: German Ministry of Science/SFB 645. Central IL-1 Receptor Signaling and Bone Mass. Funding: German-Israeli Foundation. Bone Anabolic Agents. Funding: National Institute of Health, USA. Cannabinoid Therapy for Osteoporosis. Funding: commercial sources. Oleoyl Serine and Bone Mass. Funding: US–Israel Binational Science Foundation. Depression and Bone Loss. Israel Science Foundation. Effect of Cannabinoids on Repair Processes in Bone. Funding: Israel Anti-drug Authority. Cannabinoids and Brain Function. Funding: National Institute of Health, USA.

Contents

1   **Healing of Bone Fracture: General Concepts** 1
Jona J. Sela and Itai A. Bab

Part I   Physiology of Bone Healing

2   **Cellular and Molecular Aspects of Bone Repair** 11
Itai A. Bab and Jona J. Sela

3   **Primary Mineralization** 43
Jona J. Sela

Part II   Systemic Factors in Bone Healing

4   **Anabolic Agents in Bone Repair** 51
Itai A. Bab

5   **Bone Repair in Diabetes** 59
Gail Amir

6   **Cannabinoids in Bone Repair** 67
Itai A. Bab

Part III   Bridging of Skeletal Defects and Implants

7   **Mesenchymal Stem Cells for Bone Gene Therapy** 81
Gadi Pelled, Olga Mizrahi, Nadav Kimelman-Bleich, and Dan Gazit

8   **Scaffolds in Skeletal Repair** 97
Erella Livne and Samer Srouji

9   Bone Reaction to Implants..   119
     David Kohavi

Author Index...   127

Subject Index..   151

Chapter 1
Healing of Bone Fracture: General Concepts

Jona J. Sela and Itai A. Bab

The skeleton is frequently exposed to accidental and iatrogenic insults. Bone, similar to several other tissues, portrays a marked potential for regeneration and repair. Generally, healing proceeds until a complete restoration of the osseous function and anatomy is achieved. Cellular and molecular participants are similar in healing processes of bone and other tissues of mesenchymal origin. Skeletal injury initiates a multifaceted healing process since additional non-osseous tissues are involved. In view of potential complications in the healing process, a methodological approach to expected cellular and molecular therapeutic targets is required. The study of such targets in skeletal morphogenesis reveals that the phases of bone healing display striking similarities to osseous growth and development [1–5].

Classification of the patterns of bone healing is based on a variety of events and factors that influence injury and repair. Currently, the extent of tissue loss is considered to be of critical significance. It is clear that the increase in the amount of bone loss is in direct correlation with the delay in healing. Therefore, the extent of the discontinuity between the fractured edges is accepted to serve as streamline factor for the sorting of the different types of healing. Consequently, the following two major patterns of bone repair are defined:

(a) Healing following close approximation and rigid compression of the fractured edges. This could be considered as healing in primary intention with a minimal replacement of the injured bone by intermediary tissues. The process is concluded

J.J. Sela (✉)
Laboratory of Biomineralization, Institute of Dental Sciences,
The Hebrew University Hadassah – Faculty of Dental Medicine,
P.O. Box 12272, Jerusalem 91120, Israel
e-mail: jjsela@cc.huji.ac.il

I.A. Bab
Bone Laboratory, Institute of Dental Sciences, The Hebrew University of Jerusalem,
P.O. Box 12272, Jerusalem 91120, Israel
e-mail: babi@cc.huji.ac.il

J.J. Sela and I.A. Bab (eds.), *Principles of Bone Regeneration*,
DOI 10.1007/978-1-4614-2059-0_1, © Springer Science+Business Media, LLC 2012

by a complete union between the fractured edges. Bone healing in this situation is described to occur in both lamellar and trabecular bones in instances of tight proximity of less then 0.1 mm between fractured edges with rigid stabilization. The suggested theory is that this type of healing is mediated by periosteal and endosteal tissues of the intraosseous Haversian system, marrow-derived vessels and mesenchymal cells, osteoblasts, and osteoclasts. Regeneration is characterized by bone remodeling parallel to the streamline of the osteon system. This union is formed by continuous ossification in first intention without cartilaginous or woven bone formation. The osteoclasts, engaged in necrotic bone resorption, are accompanied by the osteoblasts that form lamellar bone. Remodeling of the repaired bone is minimal in this environment consisting of minimal interfragmentary space [4]. *The concept of direct continuous bone regeneration is controversial.* It lacks basic scientific support with histological evidence in the literature. Most researchers would dispute the idea that healing could occur without formation of transient tissues between the fractured edges. It should be noted that a minimal hemorrhage is evident in all cases of trauma, and hence a blood clot, even if minimal, would develop in the fracture area serving as initial matrix for the proliferation of the involved cellular population. However, the theory on direct bone repair serves as a "scientific" justification for various orthopedic procedures. In these instances, the fracture edges are tightly pressed together. Clinical articles report a high rate of successful complete union [4]. It could be pointed out that "green stick" and "stress" fractures would probably heal in a similar manner.

(b) Healing with separated fracture edges involving intermediary tissues. These fractures are characterized by a significant gap formed between the edges with an extent of less than the diameter of the bone. Cases of such discontinuity are proven to heal regularly with artificial fixation. This type of bone healing is probably the most abundant one and is defined as healing in secondary intention (Fig. 1.1).

Clinically, fracture repair is optimized without a tight approximation of the severed edges. The course of healing constitutes several processes along the following possible stages: blood clotting, inflammatory response, granulation tissue formation, macrophage and osteoclast activity, significant bone resorption; formation of cartilaginous callus (endochondral repair) with calcification and young osseous matrix of primary bone. The continuance of the process is characterized by mineralization of the matrix.

It should be pointed out that the newly formed calcifying tissue can serve as a stabilizing but not as a weight-bearing component. Woven bone and cartilage serve as bridging templates. Complete maturation is accomplished by bone remodeling to form biomechanically compatible structures. Osseous regeneration is dependent upon several clinical issues such as location, extent of tissue loss, fracture mobility, infection, and types of reconstructive materials and systemic conditions. In addition, bone regeneration is usually accompanied by restoration of the collaterally damaged tissues, i.e., joints, cartilage, muscles, tendons, ligaments, skin, mucous membranes, bone marrow, periodontal ligament, etc. [3–5].

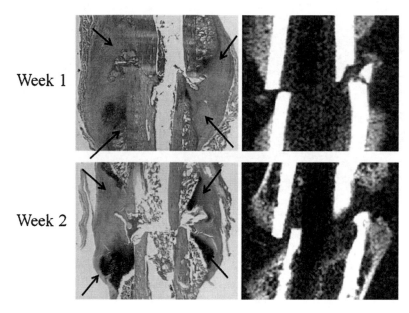

Fig. 1.1 Long bone fractures and callus in first and second weeks of healing. Note, Pairs of histological and μCT representations. *Week 1*: Callus is constructed large cartilaginous component (*arrows*), initially calcified. *Week 2*: Higher calcification (*intense violet*) and reduction of callus size

The natures of the genetic and molecular triggers that initiate and regulate the signaling pathways in the process of cellular activation in bone healing are starting to be disclosed [5–8].

Following trauma, molecules participating in fracture healing comprise proinflammatory cytokines, i.e., interleukin-1 (IL-1), interleukin-6 (IL-6), and tumor necrosis factor-α (TNF-α) that are expressed first in the inflammatory phase and later in the remodeling phase. This stage is followed by the involvement of growth and differentiation factors, including transforming growth factor-β superfamily (GDFs, BMPs, TGF-β), platelet-derived growth factor (PGDF), fibroblast growth factor (FGF), and insulin-like growth factor (IGF) that are operative few hours after the fracture time during all the reparative phase [8, 9]. Subsequently, endochondral ossification is characterized by the activities of metalloproteinases, vascular endothelial growth factors (VEGF), and angiopoietin 1 and 2. Molecules antagonist to bone morphogenetic proteins (BMPs) have been identified. Noggin, chordin, sclerostin, follistatin at extracellular setting and BAMBI (BMP and activin membrane-bound inhibitor) were observed during embryogenic development [9–11]. Canonical Wnt signaling pathway has been shown to play a role in fracture repair. This pathway, which activates Lef1/T cell factor (TCF)-dependent transcription, has emerged as a key regulator in embryonic skeletogenesis, positively regulating the osteoblasts. A significant upregulation of β-catenin was found during bone healing process A large molecular array was described to interrelate with each other and with the environment to achieve fracture repair. In this context, regulators of chemotaxis,

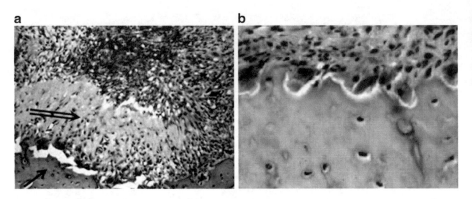

Fig. 1.2 (**a**) Fractured bone (*single arrow*), matrix with osteoblasts (*double arrow*); Note, Granulation tissue (*upper center*). (**b**) Osteoclasts in resorption lacunae (H&E staining)

mitosis, and differentiation such as Wnt, Indian hedgehog, PTHrP genes that respond to hedgehog proteins like Gli 1 and patched (Ptc), platelet-derived GF, matrix metalloproteinases (MMPs), and VEGF a, b, c, and d. Inflammatory cells produce interleukins (IL-1, IL-2, and RANKL). Tumor necrosis factor (TNF x and b) play an essential role [5, 8].

Bone injury is immediately followed by local blood clot formation that serves as a medium that allows cellular migration, proliferation, and capillary budding (Fig. 1.2). Furthermore, the clot was shown to function as a primary source for growth factors [10]. Clot formation is concomitant with the onset of the inflammatory response. At this point, expression of signaling molecules and their proposed functions include IL-1, IL-6, colony-stimulating factors, and TNF-α that play a role in initiating the repair cascade. In addition, TGF-β, PDGF, and BMP-2 expressions increase the initiation of callus formation. Recruitment of mesenchymal stem cells is associated with GDF-8 suggesting its role in controlling cellular proliferation.

It should be emphasized that impaired clotting, due to local or systemic factors, mainly coagulation disorders, anticoagulant drugs and infection, results with a major disruption of healing. The healing process continues with the resorption of the clot and its replacement by granulation tissue. This stage is characterized by an immanent cellular mobilization and vascular in growth from periosteal vessels with extensive neo-angiogenesis mediated by angiopoietins and different VEGFs. A considerable macrophage and osteoclast activity is responsible for the removal and resorption of soft and hard tissue debris by mechanisms mediated by RANKL and MCSF [12–16].

Granulation tissue represents a distinctive pattern of chronic inflammatory reaction, typical to healing in second intention. In bone repair, granulation tissue serves as a transient environment gradually replaced by an ephemeral callus of cartilage and primary bone. Granulation tissue is providing a profuse blood supply and a vehicle for cellular recruitment. At this phase, abundant undifferentiated mesenchymal cells emerge at the site of injury, proliferate, and differentiate, evidently in response to growth factors produced by the injured tissues and from the blood clot. The process

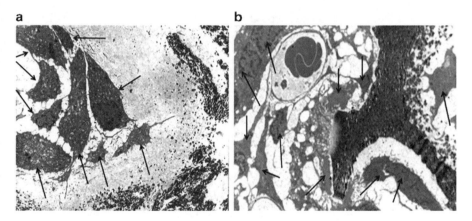

Fig. 1.3 (**a**) Osteoblasts (*arrows*) forming matrix, mineralization (*right*). (**b**) Osteoblasts (*arrows*) surrounding a bone trabecule

described involves both intramembranous and endochondral ossification (Fig. 1.3). Intramembranous ossification involves the formation of bone directly from committed osteoprogenitor cells and undifferentiated mesenchymal cells that reside mainly in the periosteum, in the Haversian tissues, and in the marrow resulting in hard callus formation [1, 4].

In endochondral ossification, chondrogenesis is assumed to be triggered by local ischemia, namely low oxygen tension, and regulated by factors such as IGF-I, PTHrP, IHH, and HIF-Iα, and mesenchymal cells differentiate into chondrocytes, producing cartilaginous matrix, which then undergoes calcification and eventually is replaced by bone. The formation of primary bone is followed by extensive remodeling until the damaged skeletal elements regain the original shape and size. As stated, these processes resemble embryonic bone formation, suggesting that fracture repair is a reiteration of normal bone development [1–5]. Regarding the molecular events, increased levels of TGF-β2, TGF-β3, and GDF-5 are associated with stem cell mobilization, chondrogenesis, endochondral and woven bone ossification. BMP-3, -4, -7, and -8 promote recruitment of cells of the osteoblastic lineage. BMP-5 and -6 rise in association with cell proliferation in intramembranous ossification. TNF-α RANKL and MCSF rise in association with mineralized cartilage resorption, apoptosis of hypertrophic chondrocytes, and matrix proteolysis. Bone remodeling coupled with osteoblast activity is associated with IL-1 and IL-6 rise, whereas RANKL and MCSF display diminished levels. Establishment of marrow is marked by diminished expression of members of the TGF-β superfamily [17]. β-Catenin signaling has been shown to play a role in fracture repair. The β-catenin signaling pathway, which activates TCF-dependent transcription, has emerged as a key regulator in embryonic skeletogenesis, positively regulating osteoblasts. A significant upregulation of β-catenin was found during bone healing process. β-Catenin functions differently at different stages of fracture repair. In early stages, precise regulation of β-catenin is required for pluripotent mesenchymal cells to differentiate to either osteoblasts or chondrocytes. Once these undifferentiated cells have become committed to the osteoblast lineage, β-catenin positively regulates osteoblasts. This is a different function for β-catenin than that has previously been reported during development. Activation of β-catenin by lithium treatment has potential to improve fracture healing, but only when used in later phases of repair after mesenchymal cells have become committed to the osteoblast lineage [18]. It is noteworthy that matrices formed during bone repair bear high similarities to those produced during embryonic limb development. Extracellular matrices are formed in healing fractures. Structural proteins, type I collagen in bone, and types II and X collagen in cartilage callus. Type III collagen is the major collagen of the fibrous matrix that forms along the periosteal surface. Type I collagen is secreted in large amounts as trabecular woven bone develops. Type V collagen is found in both fibrous tissue and bone. This type is particularly associated with blood vessels. Type II collagen is the last of the major collagens to be synthesized. Its synthesis is dependent on the mechanical conditions under which the fractures are healing particularly in instances of a large area of cartilaginous callus. Type II collagen formation is typical to mechanically unstable fractures. Type IX collagen is present throughout the large areas of cartilage. Type X is present only in calcified regions [19].

Transcription core binding factor 1 (cbfa 1) stimulates osteoblast differentiation. Additionally, bone morphogenetic proteins (BMP2, BMP3 osteogenin, BMP4, BMP7, osteogenetic protein, OP1) play a major role in bone repair [20].

Fibroblast GF2. Both fibroblast growth factors-1 (acidic FGF) and -2 (basic FGF) increase the proliferation of osteoblasts and chondrocytes in vitro and FGF-2 stimulates angiogenesis and bone formation in vivo. The application of FGF-1 or FGF-2 to normally healing fractures of the rabbit tibia did not have a significant effect on the rate of healing. Smads 1–8 serve in intracellular signaling for transforming growth factor beta (TGF-β). TGF-β was shown to stimulate bone and cartilage formation in calvarial and long bones. The effect of exogenous TGF-β2 on normally healing fractures was investigated to see if healing can be accelerated. TGF-β2 did not stimulate fracture healing under either stable or unstable mechanical conditions during the initial healing phase. Osteogenic growth peptide (OGP) was characterized in regenerating marrow. OGP-induced stimulation of bone formation in vivo suggests a role for this peptide in mediating systemic osteogenic response [15].

1.1 Distinctive Patterns of Bone Repair

1.1.1 Bone Healing Following Trauma or Marrow Injury Devoid of Fracture

This type of healing occurs in cases of bone wounds, marrow ablation, and socket healing after tooth extraction, and it is mediated by woven bone formation. Bone healing in these instances is characterized by the following stages: formation of a blood clot which is substituted by granulation tissue. The granulation tissue is replaced by woven bone. This transient tissue is remodeled to a complete restoration of the tissues in the region of the injury. In instances of bone wound healing, a full recovery is expected in accordance with the individual location of the repair. Tooth socket healing is completed after restoration of the continuity of the maxillary anatomical and histological features. In the case of bone marrow injury or ablation, reconstruction of the marrow marks the completion healing.

1.1.2 Critical Size Defect

This is defined as an extensive bone loss that prevents spontaneous healing. The gap in these cases is clinically determined to be twice the diameter of the injured bone. Due to the inability of the osseous tissue to regenerate, this condition results with repair by soft tissue callus with subsequent pseudoarthrosis usually referring to a spontaneous fractures which progress to nonunion. Experimental nonunion models in different laboratory animals have been reported with emphasis on the importance of the critical size bone defect in testing bone-regenerating materials [21–24].

References

1. Caplan AI (1987) Bone development and repair. Bioassay 6:171–175
2. Vortkamp A, Pathi S, Peretti GM, Caruso EM, Zaleske DJ, Tabin CJ (1998) Recapitulation of signals regulating embryonic bone formation during postnatal growth and in fracture repair. Mech Dev 71:65–76
3. Schneider RA, Helms JA (1998) Development and regeneration of the musculoskeletal system. Curr Opin Orthop 9:20–24
4. Shapiro F (2008) Bone development and its relation to fracture repair. The role of mesenchymal osteoblasts and surface osteoblasts. Eur Cell Mater 15:53–76, Review
5. Marzona L, Pavolini B (2009) Play and players in bone fracture healing match. Clin Cases Miner Bone Metab 6(2):159–162
6. Dimitriou R, Tsiridis E (2005) Giannoudis PV Current concepts of molecular aspects of bone healing. Injury 36:1392–1404
7. Einhorn TA (1998) The cell and molecular biology of fracture healing. Clin Orthop 355S:7–21
8. Tsiridis E, Upadhyay N, Giannoudis P (2007) Molecular aspects of fracture healing: which are the important molecules? Injury Int J Care Injured 38(S1):S11–S25
9. Cho TJ, Gerstenfeld LC, Barnes GL, Einhorn TA (2001) Cytokines and fracture healing. Curr Opin Orth 12:403–408
10. Critchlow MA, Bland YS, Ashhurst DE (1995) The effect of exogenous transforming growth factor-beta 2 on healing fractures in the rabbit. Bone 16:521–527
11. Kon T, Cho TJ, Aizawa T, Yamazaki M, Nooh N, Graves D et al (2001) Expression of osteoprotegerin, receptor activator of NF-kappa B ligand (osteoprotegerin ligand) and related proinflammatory cytokines during fracture healing. J Bone Miner Res 16:1004–1014
12. Solheim E (1998) Growth factors in bone. Int Orthop 22:410–416
13. Bland YS, Critchlow MA, Ashhurst DE (1995) Exogenous fibroblast growth factors-1 and -2 do not accelerate fracture healing in the rabbit. Acta Orthop Scand 66:543–548

14. Veillette CJH, McKee MD (2007) Growth factors – BMPs, DBMs, and buffy coat products: are there any proven differences amongst them? Injury Int J Care Injured 38(S1):S38–S48
15. Bab IA, Einhorn TA (1994) Polypeptide factors regulating osteogenesis and bone marrow repair. J Cell Biochem 55:358–365
16. Bruder SP, Fink DJ (1994) Caplan AI Mesenchymal stem cells in bone development, bone repair, and skeletal regeneration therapy. J Cell Biochem 56:283–294
17. Ai-Aql ZS, Alagl AS, Graves DT, Gerstenfeld LC, Einhorn TA (2008) Molecular mechanisms controlling bone formation during fracture healing and distraction osteogenesis. J Dent Res 87:107
18. Chen Y, Whetstone HC, Lin AC, Nadesan P, Wei Q, Poon R, Alman BA (2007) Beta-catenin signaling plays a disparate role in different phases of fracture repair: implications for therapy to improve bone healing. PLoS Med 4(7):e249
19. Ashhurst DE (1990) Collagens synthesized by healing fractures. Clin Orthop Relat Res 255:273–283
20. Reddi AH (1998) Initiation of fracture repair by bone morphogenetic proteins. Clin Orthop Relat Res 355(Suppl):S66–S72
21. Oetgen ME, Merrell GA, Troiano NW, Horowitz MC, Kacena MA (2008) Development of a femoral non-union model in the mouse. Injury 39:1119–1126
22. Bosch C, Melsen B, Vargervik K (1998) Importance of the critical-size bone defect in testing bone-regenerating materials. J Craniofac Surg 9:310–316
23. Meinel L, Fajardo R, Hofmann S, Langer R, Chen J, Snyder B, Vunjak-Novakovic G, Kaplan D (2005) Silk implants for the healing of critical size bone defects. Bone 37:688–698
24. Meinel L, Betz O, Fajardo R, Hofmann S, Nazarian A, Cory E, Hilbe M, McCool J, Langer R, Vunjak-Novakovic G, Merkle HP, Rechenberg B, Kaplan DL, Kirker-Head C (2006) Silk based biomaterials to heal critical sized femur defects. Bone 39:922–931

Part I
Physiology of Bone Healing

Chapter 2
Cellular and Molecular Aspects of Bone Repair

Itai A. Bab and Jona J. Sela

Bone healing is characterized by a series of molecular, cellular, and tissue transformations consisting of resorption and formation of hard and soft tissues. Mineralized tissue remodeling in fracture repair involves the activity of various cells, inter alia, chondroblasts, osteoblasts, osteocytes, and osteoclasts (Fig. 2.1).

Bone and cartilage are produced through a concerted generation of molecular signals that act on lineage-specific stem cells. The stem cells differentiate into various cellular phenotypes. Signal conduction via hormones, growth factors, and mechanical regulation ensures subsequent remodeling of bone and cartilage [1]. Progenitor cells are recruited from periosteal and bone marrow tissues and differentiate into matrix producing mature cells at the injured bone site. Bone is essentially a type of hard connective tissue. It is involved in the regulation of body size and height and provides structural support for skeletal muscles and physical protection of vital organs. Concomitantly, bones serve as a principal depot for calcium and phosphate minerals and the essential site of marrow tissues serving as continuous source for hematopoiesis. Bone formation by osteoblasts and resorption by osteoclasts regulate skeletal remodeling throughout the life. Osteoclasts are derived from hematopoietic stem cell (HSC) of the monocyte/macrophage lineage typically located in bone marrow and blood [1]. Bone-resorbing cells have a key role in the

I.A. Bab (✉)
Bone Laboratory, Institute of Dental Sciences,
The Hebrew University of Jerusalem, P.O. Box 12272, Jerusalem 91120, Israel
e-mail: babi@cc.huji.ac.il

J.J. Sela
Laboratory of Biomineralization, Institute of Dental Sciences,
The Hebrew University Hadassah – Faculty of Dental Medicine,
P.O. Box 12272, Jerusalem 91120, Israel
e-mail: jjsela@cc.huji.ac.il

J.J. Sela and I.A. Bab (eds.), *Principles of Bone Regeneration*,
DOI 10.1007/978-1-4614-2059-0_2, © Springer Science+Business Media, LLC 2012

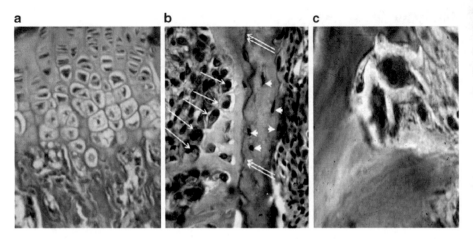

Fig. 2.1 Bone and cartilage cells. (**a**) Chondroblasts. (**b**) Osteoblasts (*arrows*) forming osteoid with Osteoblast–osteocyte transition adjacent to reversal line (*double arrows*) and osteocytes (*arrow heads*). (**c**) Osteoclasts in resorption bay

osseous healing process. Osteoblasts originate from bone marrow mesenchymal stem cells (MSCs) [2]. In healthy bone, a balance of bone formation/resorption is achieved by and large through the coordinated differentiation of these cells from their precursors. The multipotentiality of MSCs is accountable not only for the development of osteoblasts but also to a wide cellular range, including adipocytes, chondrocytes, myoblasts, and fibroblasts. MSC differentiation to the osteoblast versus adipocyte lineage has particular relevance to the maintenance of normal bone homeostasis. Accumulating evidence suggests that a shift in MSC differentiation to favor the adipocyte lineage directly contributes to imbalances in bone formation/resorption that ultimately leads to bone loss [3]. Indeed, conditions associated with bone loss such as osteoporosis and glucocorticoid excess coincides with increased bone marrow adiposity [2, 3]. The balance between adipogenic and osteogenic differentiation is regulated by ligands such as bone morphogenetic proteins (BMPs) and the osteogenic growth peptide (OGP) and receptor/transcription factor PPARγ [4, 5]. However, a multitude of regulators, including neurotransmitters and peptides, hormones, growth factors, and transcription factors are involved in the regulation of the complex and finely tuned process of osteoblast differentiation. During bone healing, the adipogenic–osteoblastogenic balance of stem cell differentiation is completely shifted toward the chondrocyte/osteoblast cell line [4–7]. Cartilage and/or bone matrices serve as provisional bridging of the fracture gap providing mechanically functional components. The coordinated production of these skeletal tissues requires timely recruitment of the progenitor cells at the site and their differentiation into chondroblasts and/or osteoblasts. Disturbances in any one of these events can have a hindering effect on bone repair.

2.1 Osteoblasts

The osteoblasts produce and regulate bone matrix and mineralization during development, remodeling, and regeneration (Fig. 2.2).

Osteoblasts arise from MSCs that develop according to a well-documented course of gene expression, progressing from osteoblastic commitment to proliferation, and final morpho-differentiation. Bone formation and repair by osteoblasts are the basis of healing of skeletal injuries and restorative procedures (Fig. 2.3).

2.2 Osteocytes

The osteocyte is the mature form of the osteoblast.

Osteoblasts and osteocytes [3, 6] produce connections with the existing embedded cells (Fig. 2.4). While becoming engulfed in the matrix, the cells are referred to as osteoid–osteocytes [7].

Mineralization of the matrix completes the osteocytic maturation. The osteocyte embedded in mineralized matrix is the stationary resident responsible for function and metabolism of bone tissue (Fig. 2.5). Osteocytes make up more than 90–95% of all bone cells in the adult skeleton.

Osteoblasts compose less than 5% and osteoclasts less than 1%. Osteocytes are viable for years, even decades, whereas osteoblasts live lifetimes of weeks and osteoclasts of days. The unique feature of osteocytes is the formation of long processes that connect through minute tubules in the bone matrix with one another and

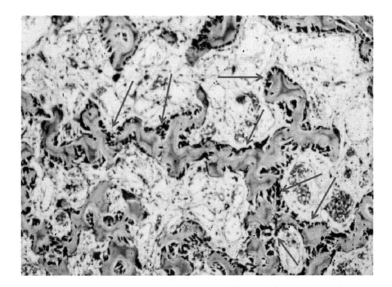

Fig. 2.2 Osteoblasts (*arrows*) aligned along primary bone surfaces

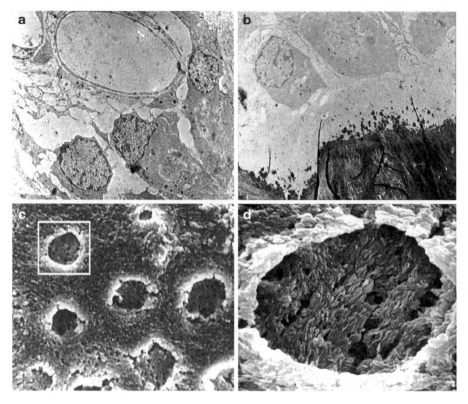

Fig. 2.3 Electron micrographs of different osteoblastic features. (**a**) Osteoblasts adjacent to blood capillary. (**b**) Osteoblasts adjacent to Calcifying front (TEM). (**c**) Osteoblastic lacunae on surface (SEM). (**d**) Higher magnification of the square in C, an osteocytic lacunae (SEM)

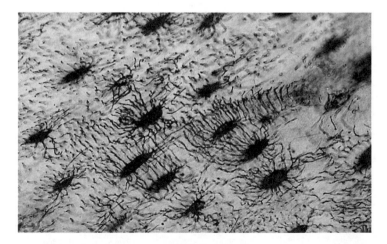

Fig. 2.4 Osteocytes and cellular processes demonstrated by impregnation methodology

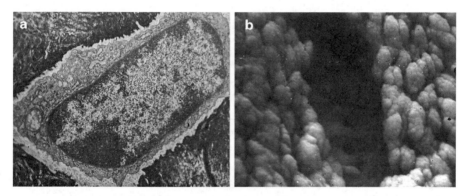

Fig. 2.5 Electron micrographs demonstrating osteocytic features. (**a**) Osteocyte embedded in mineralized matrix (TEM). (**b**) Osteocytic lacuna (SEM)

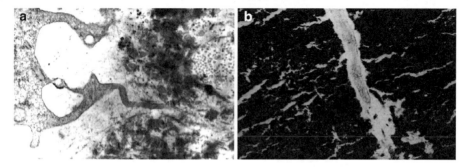

Fig. 2.6 Osteocytic processes (TEM). (**a**) Osteocyte with processes embedded in the mineralized matrix (horizontal). (**b**) Osteocytic process traversing in canaliculus in heavily calcified bone (perpendicular)

with cells on the bone surface. These processes have been shown to extend into the bone marrow [4] (Fig. 2.6).

Osteocytes send signals of both bone resorption and bone formation. It has been proposed that at death phases, osteocytes send signals initiating resorption [5, 8]. Recently, it has been shown that sclerostin, a highly expressed protein in osteocytes, targets osteoblasts to inhibit bone formation [9]. It has been suggested that osteocytes act as orchestrators, directing both osteoclast and osteoblast activity in bone remodeling. A major issue in the understanding of bone regulation concerns the probable sensing of mechanical strains by the osteocyte. It is thought that cells on the bone surface (lining cells, osteoblasts) are subjected to substrate strain, whereas osteocytes "sense" mechanical strain due to fluid flow shear stress. Osteocytes when compared to osteoblasts are more responsive to fluid flow shear stress than to other form of mechanical strain, such as substrate stretching [10]. It has been proposed that osteocytes sense shear stress mainly along their cellular processes and the cell body. Osteocytic deformation in vitro correlates with the extent of shear stress, which in turn is in direct relationship with a biological response manifested in prostaglandin release.

PKD1 and 2 are known to have mechano-sensory functions in the kidney and were shown to be expressed in bone. Deletion of PKD1 function results in animals with a bone defect [11]. In a search for markers highly expressed on osteocytes, the E11/gp38 molecule was found first in MLO-Y4 osteocyte-like cells and also in early embedding osteocytes in bone but not in cells on the bone surface [12, 13]. E11/gp38 is a 40 kDa transmembrane protein thought to play a role in the formation of cellular processes in various cell types. Cells with extensive cellular projections, such as podocytes and type1 alveolar lung cells, etc., express high amounts of E11/gp38. This membrane molecule appears to play a role in dendrite elongation, as MLO-Y4 cells subjected to fluid flow shear stress elongate their processes, and this elongation was blocked by siRNA [13]. Conditional deletion of this gene results in neonatal lethality due to lung defects [14]. In vivo loading induced elevation in both gene and protein expression of E11/gp38, not only near the bone surface but also in deeply embedded bone in response to loading [13]. It was not clear why a molecule proposed to have a role in dendrite formation would be increased in deeply embedded osteocytes-cells thought to have their dendrites stationary and tethered to the walls of their canaliculi [15, 16]. However, dynamic imaging of viable calvarial bone has shown that osteocytes can extend and retract their cell processes [17]. This suggests that E11/gp38 could be involved in the extension of dendrites in osteocytes embedded in bone in response to load. Observations using static data limit our thinking and ability to form more accurate and novel hypotheses, whereas dynamic imaging has opened a whole new area for investigation. Cellular and molecular mechanisms involved in osteoblast formation are of major significance for the progress of curative procedures. Selective expression of master transcriptional regulators is responsible for lineage commitment of MSCs. The myogenic path is regulated by MyoD (myosin dictyostelium); PPARγ (peroxisome proliferator activated receptor gamma) promotes adipogenesis; Sox9 (SRY-sex determining region Y-box 9) and Runx2 (Runt-related transcription factor 2) are responsible for chondrocytic and osteoblast differentiation, respectively [8–11, 18]. Lineage commitment of osteoprogenitors is followed by a proliferative stage, characterized by the production of proteins such as histones, fibronectin, type I collagen c-Fos (antisense oligonucleotide), c-Jun (N-terminal kinases), and p21 (cyclin-dependent kinase inhibitor 1) [12]. Following division, cellular transition expresses genes such as alkaline phosphatase, bone sialoprotein, and type I collagen, producing osteogenic extracellular matrix. Concomitantly the osteoblasts express genes engaged in mineralization of the extracellular matrix such as osteocalcin, osteopontin, and collagenase [13]. Transcription factors including Runx2, Osx (osterix, osteoblast-specific transcription factor), SMADs, TCF/LEF (transcription factor/lymphoid enhancer factor), NFATc1 (nuclear factor of activated T-cells, cytoplasmic, calcineurin-dependent 1), Twist (twist homolog 1), AP-1 (adaptor-related protein complex 1), and ATF4 (activating transcription factor 4) regulate the program of gene expression and cellular differentiation. Notably, micro-RNAs (miRs) have been identified as regulators of osteoblast gene expression. The mechanistic control of gene expression by cofactors such as acetyltransferases and histone deacetylases (HDACs) has been identified. Numerous transcription factors and epigenetic

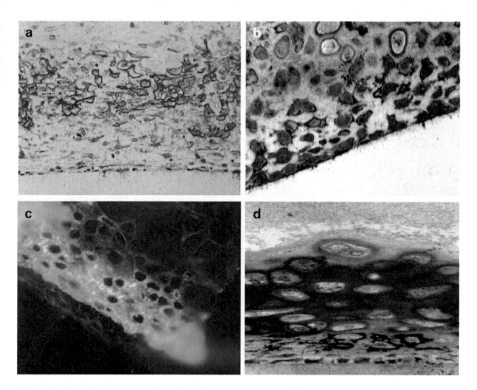

Fig. 2.7 Osteoblasts producing mineralizing matrix in diffusion chamber cultures of MSCs. (**a**) Osteoblast cell membranes stained red with histochemical reaction for alkaline phosphatase. (**b**) Autoradiograph showing distribution of PTH receptors. (**c**) Immunohistochemical staining of collagen type I in osteoblast layer. (**d**) Periosteoblast mineral deposition demonstrated by Von Kossa staining

co-regulators are involved in the genesis of the osteoblast and in the mechanisms that determine the functions as regulators of gene expression (Fig. 2.7, Table 2.1).

Runx2 is often depicted as main regulator of osteoblast-genesis [14] (Table 2.1). It operates during induction, proliferation, and maturation of osteoblasts and controls expression of a range of genes. Haplo-insufficiency of Runx2 causes skeletal abnormalities, delayed ossification of skull-bones, cleidocranial dysostosis, and dental defects. Homozygous mutation of Runx2 is lethal in mice due to a complete lack of mineralized bone [11, 15, 18]. Runx2 expression is poorly correlated with expression of its target genes, indicating that Runx2 activity is regulated by additional factors. In fact, Runx2 is subject to posttranslational regulation by phosphorylation, acetylation, and ubiquitination. In addition to its Runt-class DNA-binding motif, Runx2 protein contains multiple domains that mediate either transcriptional activation or repression through associations with co-activators or co-repressors [16, 17]. These various modes of control enable Runx2 to function as a master

Table 2.1 Sequential marker-gene expression in osteoblast differentiation

Stromal stem cell	Osteoprogenitor	Pre-osteoblast	Osteoblast	Osteocyte
Sca-1	Runx2	Runx2	Runx2	Runx2
Stro-1	Osx	Osx	Osx	Osx
	COL-1	COL-1	COL-1	COL-1
		TNSALP	TNSALP	TNSALP
		PTHRc	PTHRc	PTHRc
			OCN	OCN
				SOST
				DMP1

regulator, integrating diverse signals to activate or repress transcription in a precise spatiotemporal manner and in response to changing physiological needs.

Further co-activators of Runx2 function comprise histone acetyltransferases, p300, CBP, PCAF, MOZ, and MORF [19, 20]. These can add acetyl groups to lysine residues of histone and non-histone target proteins, which modifies protein function by a variety of mechanisms including altered protein–protein interaction and altered protein stability. In the case of nucleosomal histones, acetylation is associated with a more open chromatin structure, recruitment of bromo-domain proteins, and increased transcriptional activity at a locus, while histone deacetylation catalyzed by HDACs is correlated with chromatin condensation and transcriptional repression. The interaction between Runx2 and HDACs is based on the observation that HDAC inhibitors reduce the activities of various Runx2 repression domains [21]. A candidate gene approach confirmed that HDAC6 binds Runx2 and represses its activity. Furthermore, Runx2 is functionally inhibited by HDAC3, HDAC4, HDAC5, and HDAC7 [22–27]. HDAC proteins are known to form large multicomponent repressive complexes composed of cofactors such as NCor, SMRT, and Sin3a, as well as multiple HDACs. It remains poorly understood how these complexes participate in the regulation of Runx2 activity, although it has been shown that Runx2 target gene expression is repressed by HDACs through multiple distinct mechanisms and in response to various osteogenic signals such as BMP2 and PTH. Runx2 was shown to recruit HDAC3 to the BSP promoter, where it represses transcription by deacetylating histones [27]. Runx2 protein is subject to proteolysis in response to Smurf1 (SMAD-specific E3 ubiquitin protein ligase 1) and Schnurri-WWP1 ubiquitin ligases [27–36] (Schnurri, Mammalian Homolog of the *Drosophila* Zinc Finger Adapter Protein Shn). BMP2 protects Runx2 from Smurf1-catalyzed proteolysis by stimulating Runx2 acetylation through a SMAD-dependent mechanism [23]. Runx2 acetylation by p300 is counteracted by HDAC4 and HDAC5, which remove the acetyl groups from Runx2, thus promoting Runx2 ubiquitin-mediated proteolysis (Interestingly, estrogen receptor-related receptor γ, an orphan nuclear receptor whose expression in osteoblasts is stimulated by BMP2, competes with p300 (E1A binding protein p300) for binding to Runx2 and inhibits BMP2-induced osteoblast formation [37]. Runx2 recruits both HDAC6 [21] and HDAC7 [22] to chromatin, which repress Runx2 target gene transcription. However, the mechanism of this repression is still incompletely understood. Inhibitors of deacetylase enzymatic activity facilitate repression by HDAC6 [21], whereas HDAC7 represses Runx2 through a not yet revealed mechanism that does not require its deacetylase domain or catalytic activity [22]. BMP2 activates protein kinase D 1 (PKD1), which phosphorylates HDAC7, leading to a transient export of HDAC7 from the nucleus, and freeing Runx2 from HDAC7's repression [38]. HDACs 4, 5, and 7 can be exported from the nucleus in response to the same set of protein kinases, yet they exhibit different subcellular distributions and respond differently to BMP2 stimulation in osteoblast-like cells [38]. Parathyroid hormone (PTH) regulates skeletal physiology by stimulation of Runx2 interactions with acetyltransferases. PTH is a strong inducer of matrix metallopeptidase, MMP-13 transcription in osteoblasts [39, 40]. Stimulation of these cells with PTH leads to a protein kinase A-dependent binding of p300 to Runx2 on the MMP-13 promoter, resulting in increased histone acetylation and gene transcription [41]. PTH also regulates Runx2 activity through other mechanisms such as phosphorylation [42] and promotes interactions with adaptor-related protein complex 1, AP-1 transcription factors [43, 44]. Finally, PTH decreases Runx2 protein stability by ubiquitin-mediated proteolysis, limiting PTH stimulation of osteoblastic genes [36].

Osterix: (Osx, also known as Sp7) is a Runx2-induced transcription factor expressed in osteogenic cell progenitors, committing them to the osteoblast, rather than chondroblast lineage [45]. Osx-null mice die at birth due to lack of mineralized skeletons. Bones formed by intramembranous ossification are entirely non-mineralized, while endochondral bones exhibit regions of mineralized cartilage, indicating that Osx functions specifically in osteoblasts. Despite its evident importance in bone formation, relatively little is known about regulation of Osx expression, its functional partners, or its direct target genes. Osx expression was believed to be downstream of Runx2, because Runx2 expression is normal in Osx-null mice, while Osx expression is absent in Runx2-knockout mice [45]. This was confirmed through characterization of a Runx2-binding element in the Osx gene promoter [46]. Osterix activation of the Col1A1 (collagen, type 1, alpha 1) promoter is enhanced by binding of NFATc1 to Osx, an interaction that is disrupted by calcineurin [47]. Another function of osterix is as an inhibitor of canonical Wnt signaling by inhibiting DNA binding of transcription factors [48] (Table 2.1).

ATF4 (activating transcription factor 4): RSK2 is a ribosomal serine/threonine kinase mutated in Coffin–Lowry Syndrome, a disorder that includes various skeletal abnormalities. The positive role of ATF4 on osteoblast formation was recognized with the findings that it is a substrate for the RSK2 kinase and ATF4-deficiency decreased bone formation [49], while forced accumulation of ATF4 induced osteoblastic gene expression in non-osseous cells [50]. ATF4 forms a complex with Runx2 at the osteocalcin promoter to increase osteocalcin *transcription* [51]. The transcriptional activity of this complex is furthered by PTH signaling and by associations with C-EBP (CAAT-enhancer binding protein) and the TFIIAγ (General Transcription Factor IIA-Gamma) [52–54]. (CCAAT is the abbreviation for cytidine–cytidine–adenosine–adenosine–thymidine.) Interestingly, ATF4 in osteoblasts was recently found to regulate energy metabolism through decreased insulin production and insulin responsiveness via altered osteocalcin and leptin endocrine signaling pathways [55, 56].

2.3   SMADs (A Combination of Two Abbreviations, SMA and MAD)

SMAD proteins are homologs of both *Caenorhabditis elegans* protein SMA and the drosophila protein, mothers against DPP = DecaPentaPlegic MAD. The BMP and TGFβ families of growth factors have long been recognized as vital regulators of skeletal physiology. TGFβ or BMP signaling leads to phosphorylation and nuclear translocation of receptor-activated SMADs (rSMADs). These interact directly with the DNA and associate with other transcription factors to regulate gene transcription. rSMADs direct mesenchymal cells into the osteoblast lineage through induction of Runx2 expression[57]. They also interact with the Runx2 protein to synergistically regulate transcription [57–61]. The SMAD-interaction domain in Runx2 has been identified and is continuous with the nuclear matrix targeting sequence, which is necessary for Runx2 function [60–62]. SMADs are inactivated by Smurf-directed ubiquitination, resulting in their proteolytic degradation. An interesting feedback loop between BMP/SMAD/Runx2 signaling is indicated by recent studies which showed that BMPs act through Runx2 to induce expression of SMAD6, an inhibitory SMAD protein that represses BMP signaling [63]. SMAD6 stimulates Runx2 ubiquitination and degradation by Smurf1 [64]. This process would be a potential mechanism to prevent excess BMP/Runx2-mediated osteogenesis (Table 2.1).

NFATc1/Calcineurin: NFATc1 (nuclear factor of activated T-cells) is a transcription factor that plays a central role in osteoclast formation and in T-cell development [65]. In unstimulated cells, NFATc1 is highly phosphorylated and localized to the cytoplasm. Intracellular calcium signaling activates the phosphatase calcineurin, which dephosphorylates NFATc1, permitting its nuclear import and NFATc1-mediated gene expression. Given the importance of NFATc1 in osteoclastogenesis, it would be expected that administration of calcineurin inhibitors would suppress resorption and increase bone mass; however, calcineurin inhibitors actually result in ostepenia. Koga et al. resolved this paradox by showing that in addition to inhibiting osteoclasts, calcineurin inhibitors blocked osteoblast maturation and mineralization by preventing a previously unknown synergy between NFATc1 and osterix in osteoblasts [47]. In a subsequent study, Choo et al. showed that overexpressed constitutively active (nuclear) NFATc1 inhibited MC3T3 E1 osteoblast differentiation in vitro and reduced expression of osteocalcin as a result of inhibited TCF/LEF transcriptional activity, which was due to sustained recruitment of HDAC3 and decreased histone acetylation at the proximal osteocalcin promoter [26].

Twist: Twist is a basic helix-loop-helix transcription factor that regulates differentiation of multiple cell types. Heterozygosity for Twist-1 in mice or humans results in premature fusion of the skull sutures, suggesting that Twist antagonizes osteoblast formation [66–70]. One mechanism through which Twist-1 acts to impair osteoblastogenesis is by binding to the Runx2 DNA-binding domain and inhibiting its ability to bind DNA [69]. Twist also inhibits BMP/SMAD responsive transcription by forming a complex with Smad4 and HDAC1 [70].

AP-1: The AP-1 class of transcription factors is composed of heterodimers of Fos-related factors (c-Fos, Fra1, Fra2, and FosB) and Jun proteins (c-Jun, JunB, and JunD). Multiple Fos and Jun proteins are highly expressed in proliferating osteoprogenitors. Their expression decreases during differentiation such that Fra2 and JunD are the primary AP-1 components present in mature osteoblasts [71]. Targeted deletion and transgenic overexpression strategies have been used to examine the role of individual Fos and Jun proteins in mice. Deletion of c-Fos had little effect on bone formation [72], while its overexpression led to osteosarcomas [73]. Fra1 and ΔFosB (an alternative splice variant of FosB) overexpressing mice exhibit enhanced osteoblast formation [74, 75], while deletion of Fra1 or JunB reduced bone mass. Recent work by Chang et al. demonstrates that inhibition of NF-κB signaling specifically in differentiated osteoblasts promotes bone formation through increased Fra1 expression [76]. These observations indicate that AP-1 proteins promote bone formation. In contrast, deletion of JunD increased bone mass, apparently by increasing expression of Fra1, Fra2, and c-Jun, suggesting that JunD represses expression of other AP-1 proteins in osteoblasts [77]. A number of direct targets of AP-1 in osteoblasts have been identified, and include the osteocalcin, collagenase-3 (MMP13), bone sialoprotein, and alkaline phosphatase promoters [78]. At these promoters, AP-1 physically and functionally interacts with other transcription factors such as the vitamin D receptor and Runx2 to regulate gene expression. Yet another layer of complexity to AP-1 signaling involves alternative protein isoforms. As mentioned above, ΔFosB, which is a splice variant of FosB that lacks the amino-terminus, promotes osteoblast formation through incompletely understood mechanisms. Translational initiation of the ΔFosB mRNA from an internal methionine can produce a further truncated protein, known as Δ2ΔFosB, which lacks any known transcriptional activation domains, yet enhances osteoblast formation by increasing BMP/SMAD signaling [78].

Tcf7/Lef1 TranscriptionFactors: Tcf7 proteins and Lef1 are high mobility group proteins best known as nuclear effectors of canonical Wnt signaling. Activation of the canonical Wnt signal transduction pathway stabilizes β-catenin, which translocates to the nucleus and associates with Tcf/Lef1 transcription factors, displacing HDACs and other co-repressors while recruiting additional co-activators to stimulate gene expression [79–83]. Tcf7 (also known as Tcf1), Tcf7L2 (Tcf4), and Lef1 are expressed in osseous cells [84–87]. Although Tcfs are functionally redundant in some instances, emerging evidence demonstrates distinct roles for Tcf7/Lef1 factors in osteoblasts. Expression of a mutated and constitutively activated version of the Tcf7/Lef1 co-activator, β-catenin, in osteoblasts using the (2.3)ColIA promoter stimulated osteoprotegerin (OPG) expression, leading to decreased osteoclastogenesis and bone resorption, but had little effect on osteoblast formation [84]. Conversely, Tcf7 knockout mice showed decreased OPG expression, enhanced osteoclast activity, and increased resorption [84]. Lef1 also contributes to osteoblast function. Lef1+/− female mice exhibited reduced osteoblast activity resulting in decreased bone mass [88], while homozygous Lef1−/− mice show reduced body size and die by 2 weeks of age [86]. Lef1 expression decreases during osteoblast differentiation and overexpression of Lef1 inhibited differentiation and expression of late osteoblast markers, indicating that Lef1 inhibits late stages of osteoblastogenesis

[85, 89]. Subsequent work by Hoeppner et al. identified an alternative variant of Lef1, Lef1ΔN, which lacks the N-terminal β-catenin binding domain [90]. Lef1ΔN expression increases during differentiation and in response to BMP signaling and Runx2, and leads to accelerated osteoblast formation. Likewise, although Runx2 expression is directly enhanced through canonical Wnt signaling through TCF-7 [91], Runx2's transcriptional activity is repressed by binding to Tcf/Lef transcription factors in osteoblasts, providing a novel means for feedback between Wnts signaling and Runx2 [85]. Wnt signaling is believed to act downstream of BMP signaling in the differentiation of pre-osteoblastic cells, as induction of osteoblasts by Wnt3a or activated β-catenin is independent of BMP signaling, whereas attenuated Wnt signaling impairs BMP2-induced expression [92–94]. Wnt-responsive transcription in osteoblasts is also antagonized by FGF signaling, through decreased expression of frizzleds and TCF/LEFs [95] (TCF/LEF—T-cell factor/lymphoid enhancer factor). Together, these studies demonstrate functional complexity within the TCF/LEF family and illustrate some of the opportunities for regulatory crosstalk to integrate diverse signals and modulate gene expression in osteoblasts.

ZFP, Zinc FingerProteins: Two major families of zinc finger transcription factors are the Kruppel-like factors (KLFs) and specificity proteins (Sps). Members of both groups participate in regulation of gene expression in osteoblasts through interactions with other transcription factors at target gene promoters. Zfp521, a KLF protein, is expressed in osteoblast precursors, osteoblasts, and osteocytes, as well as chondrocytes [96]. Its expression increases during osteoblast differentiation and in response to PTHrP, while BMP2 decreases ZFP521 levels. ZFP521 binds to Runx2 and antagonizes Runx2 gene transactivation, and overexpression of ZFP521 in in vitro osteoblast cultures impairs their differentiation. These observations indicate an inhibitory role for Zfp521 in osteoblasts. Unexpectedly, mice overexpressing ZFP521 in osteoblasts, under control of the OG2 osteocalcin promoter element, exhibit increased bone mass, even though isolated calvarial osteoblasts from these mice show impaired osteoblastic differentiation. The authors speculated that this difference may stem from the OG2 promoter not being expressed until relatively late in osteoblastogenesis. The Sp family of transcription factors is ubiquitously expressed (with the exception of Osx, which is also known as Sp7), and is involved with both basal and induced gene expression. Sp1 cooperates with ETS transcription factors at the Runx2 P1 promoter to stimulate transcription of Runx2 [97]. In osteoblasts, Sp1 and Sp3 cooperate with TGFβ-responsive SMADs to induce the β5 integrin promoter [98]. Similarly, Sp1 cooperates with Runx2 to mediate PTH-induction of the matrix gla protein promoter, while Sp3 is an inhibitor of this promoter [99].

2.4   Regulation of Osteoblast Gene Expression by MicroRNAs

Progress in the understanding of the regulation of osteogenesis involves the role of miRs. Short noncoding RNAs, range from 18 to 25 nucleotides, which regulate gene expression by binding to the 3′-UTR of mRNAs for specific target genes and inhibiting gene expression by either promoting degradation of the target mRNAs or inhibiting their translation [100]. Many of these miRs inhibit osteogenesis through repression of osteoblastic genes. In an important study, Li et al. identified a novel mechanism through which BMP-2 promotes osteoblastogenesis [101]. By RNA expression profiling, they identified a set of 22 miRs whose expression was reduced by BMP2 stimulation of C2C12 mesenchymal cells. These miRs are predicted to inhibit a range of pro-osteogenic factors; hence, reduced levels of these miRs should enhance expression of osteogenic genes. Osteoblastic proliferation is inhibited by miR-125b, which inhibits the ErbB2 receptor tyrosine kinase [101]. Two miRs that inhibit expression of Dlx5 (distal-less homeobox 5) in pre-osteoblasts have been identified [102]. MiR-29a and miR-29c are expressed in response to canonical Wnt signaling and inhibit expression of the extracellular matrix protein Osteonectin, which is important in numerous processes in skeletal physiology [103]. Not all miRs are functional inhibitors of osteoblastogenesis. TGFβ signaling inhibits osteo-genesis, and MiR-210 acts as a positive regulator of osteoblastic differentiation by inhibiting expression of ACVR1B (activin receptor 1B) for TGFβ [104].

2.5   Chondroblast

The process of fracture healing exhibits often a high similarity to endochondral ossification. This has been confirmed by numerous histological, cellular, and molec-ular studies. Consequently, a description of the cells involved in this process and their regulation are briefly reviewed. Since the body of information on the cellular and molecular processes in growth plate cartilage (Fig. 2.8) is substantially greater, this process is described below as a paradigm highly relevant to fracture healing.

In endochondral ossification, progenitor cells present in the resting zone serve as a reservoir for the proliferative cellular zone. Further maturation is characterized by termination of cell division and further differentiation into prehypertrophic and later to hypertrophic chondrocytes [105–108] (Fig. 2.9).

Both proliferating and hypertrophic chondrocytes secrete extracellular matrices that typically contain collagen type II and type X, respectively. The extracellular matrix in the hypertrophic cell zone mineralizes. Following resorption by chondro-clasts/osteoclasts, the cartilage is replaced by trabecullar bone [106, 108–110].

Although critically affected by growth hormone, the regulation of endochondral ossification has been attributed primarily to mechanisms intrinsic to the cartilage [105, 111]. The cartilage maturation and eventual resorption and replacement are associated with structural changes such as reduced heights of the proliferative and hypertrophic cell zones, as well as reduced hypertrophic cell size and column den-sity [112]. It has been suggested that this decline occurs since the progenitor cells have a definitive proliferative capacity that is gradually exhausted [105, 112, 113]. The cartilaginous intrinsic paracrine factors that regulate chondrocyte proliferation, differentiation, and senescence are insulin-like growth factors I (IGF-I), Indian

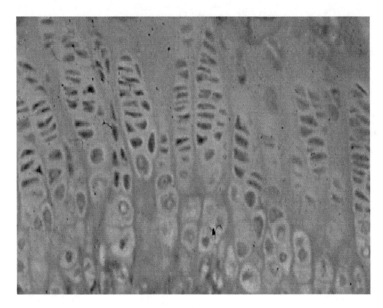

Fig. 2.8 Growth plate cartilage; note, typical palisading chondrocytes. Proliferating cells (*upper*). Hypertrophic differentiated cells (*lower*)

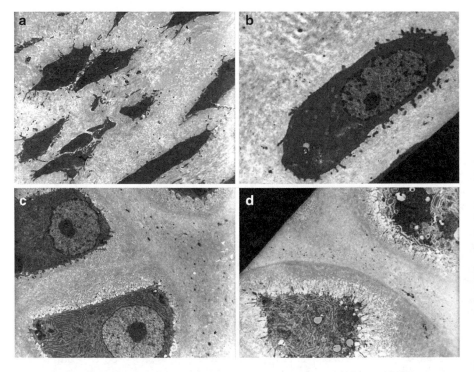

Fig. 2.9 Electron micrographs of growth plate chondroblasts. (**a**) Proliferative zone. (**b**) Prehypertrophic differentiation. (**c**) Hypertrophic chondrocytes. (**d**) Apoptotic chondrocytes

hedgehog (Ihh), PTH-related protein (PTHrP), fibroblast growth factors (FGF), transforming growth factor β (TGFβ), and BMPs.

IGF-I: The main cartilage intrinsic regulator is IGF-I, which is expressed in proliferating chondrocytes and to a lesser extent in hypertrophic chondrocytes [114]. It should be noted that exogenously administered IGF-I can markedly improve linear skeletal growth, supporting a suggested role for circulating IGF-I [105, 115].

IGF-Binding Proteins (IGFBPs): The cellular availability of IGF-I is also regulated by the IGFBPs, a family of proteins with high affinity especially for IGF-I. IGFBP-2, -3, -4, and -5 are present in all layers of the osteogenic cartilage, with IGFBP-3, -4, and -5 expressions being reduced in hypertrophic chondrocytes. IGFBPs are regulated by IGF-I and to a lesser extent by IGF-II [116].

Ihh: Indian hedgehog is a member of the family of hedgehog (HH) proteins that includes also sonic HH (SHH) and desert HH (DHH). The HH signal is received and transduced via a specific receptor complex composed of patched (PTCH) and smoothened (SMOH) transmembrane proteins [117]. Ihh is expressed in the prehypertrophic cells that have just stopped proliferating [118–121]. Its main action in the osteogenic cartilage is through the regulation of PTH-related peptide (PTHrP) [118–120]. Ihh appears to be both necessary and sufficient for PTHrP expression [122]. It inhibits hypertrophic chondrocyte differentiation, and thereby delays the mineralization of the cartilage matrix and its resorption. Ihh regulates cartilage development through PTHrP-independent pathways as well. Ihh stimulates differentiation of periarticular to columnar chondrocytes thereby regulating column length independently of PTHrP [119, 121, 123].

PTHrP: This is an auto/paracrine factor [118] that binds to and activates the PTH/PTHrP receptor, which is also activated by PTH [124], a G protein-coupled receptor. In osteogenic cartilage, PTHrP mRNA is expressed by perichondrial cells and proliferating chondrocytes in the periarticular region [122]. The PTH/PTHrP receptor is expressed in proliferating/prehypertrophic chondrocytes. Its activation delays maturation thus ensuring a supply of proliferating chondrocytes, which is essential for skeletal growth and repair [125]. Cells at a distance from the source of PTHrP withdraw from the cell cycle and begin terminal differentiation. PTHrP appears to promote chondrocyte proliferation and delays differentiation by several mechanisms [121, 125]. It inhibits production of p57, an inhibitor of cyclin-dependent protein kinases. It also regulates phosphorylation of the transcription factor Sox9, a master transcription factor in chondrogenesis. Sox9 phosphorylation increases its transcriptional efficiency and decreases terminal differentiation. PTHrP also decreases the production of Runx2 [125, 126], a transcription factor essential for osteoblast-specific gene expression and for bone formation. Recent experiments have shown that Runx2 is expressed in the prehypertrophic and hypertrophic zones of embryonic mouse cartilages and plays a role in chondrocyte maturation. [122, 125, 126].

The Ihh-PTHrP circuit is regulated by IGF-I. Lack of IGF-I alters this circuit, dissociating the regulation of Ihh and PTHrP, which results in downregulation of Ihh expression and upregulation of PTHrP expression [127]. In the growth plate,

IGF-I deficiency results in an elevated, abnormally distributed, PTHrP expression in proliferative and hypertrophic chondrocytes. This would be expected to delay the rate of differentiation of chondrocytes, and delay mineralization, similar to overexpression of PTHrP in transgenic mice [127].

FGF: The FGFs comprise a family of secreted proteins that form a trimolecular complex by binding to one of four high affinity FGF receptors (FGFRs) and heparan sulfate proteoglycans [128–132]. All FGFRs are expressed in the osteogenic cartilage. FGFR3 has gained more attention than the other FGFRs. It is a master inhibitor of chondrocyte proliferation and growth [118, 132, 133]. Mutations in FGFR3 lead to short stature syndromes [118, 132, 133]. This effect of FGFR3 signaling involves direct action on chondrocytes as well as suppression of Ihh expression [120]. The FGFRs are activated by FGF-1,-2,-7,-17,-18,-19, and -22 [132].

Wnt Proteins (Wingless-type MMTV Integration Site Family) (MMTV abbreviation of Mouse Mammary Tumor Virus): Wnt proteins are powerful secreted signaling factors that regulate a number of developmental processes [123, 134]. The vertebrate Wnt family currently comprises 20 members. Wnt proteins act by binding to Frizzled and low-density lipoprotein receptor-related protein cell surface receptors. Upon Wnt binding, Frizzled receptors transduce signals via the β-catenin-LEF/TCF pathway, Ca2-calmodulin–PKC pathway, or JNK-dependent pathway [134]. Depending on the developmental stage, disruption of the canonical β-catenin pathway either blocks chondrocyte hypertrophy and endochondral ossification (early stages) or stimulates hypertrophy and ossification (later stages) [134]. The Wnt family member mainly implicated in growth regulation is Wnt9a, acting as a temporal and spatial positive regulator of Ihh [123].

TGFβ: TGFβ-related proteins form a large family of secreted molecules including, among others, TGFβs, activins, and BMPs [106, 109, 135]. These molecules form either homodimers or heterodimers, and exert their activity through type I and type II serine/threonine kinase receptors. ALK5/TGFβRI and TGFβRII are expressed in proliferating and hypertrophic chondrocytes and in the perichondrium [106, 109, 135]. TGFβ is secreted by chondrocytes and stimulates PTHrP production in perichondrial cells [109]. Disrupting the TGFβ signaling pathway (SMAD 3) lead to progressive cartilage abnormalities, including premature hypertrophy of growth plate chondrocytes and disorganization of the growth plate columns resulting in decreased longitudinal growth [109, 136].

BMPs: In the osteogenic cartilage, most of the BMP expression is found in the perichondrium (BMP-2, -3, -4, -5, and -7). In addition, BMP-2 and -6 are present in hypertrophic chondrocytes and BMP-7 in proliferative chondrocytes [118]. The BMPs are positive modulators of chondrocyte proliferation and negatively regulators of chondrocyte terminal differentiation [118, 137]. BMP-6 accelerates calcified matrix deposition, thus being involved in the cartilage-to-bone transition [138]. The type I BMP receptors exhibit characteristic expression patterns in the cartilage. BMPR1A is highly expressed in the perichondrium and in proliferating and hypertrophic chondrocytes. BMPR1B is found throughout the cartilage

[137, 139]. The type II BMP receptor is also expressed throughout the cartilage. BMPR1A has been implicated in the differentiation of proliferating chondrocytes toward hypertrophic chondrocytes [140]. BMPs interact with the IHH/PTHrP pathway by promoting Ihh expression by prehypertrophic chondrocytes and can therefore increase the proliferation of chondrocytes [124, 137]. IHH controls BMP levels, operating in a positive feedback loop [137].

Hypoxia: The osteogenic cartilage is largely avascular, resulting in low O_2 tension. There is an O_2 gradient with lowest levels of O_2 in chondrocytes of the core hypertrophic zone [140, 141]. The hypoxic signals are transmitted to the cells by prolyl hydroxylases (PHDs), which are O_2 sensor proteins found in chondrocytes [141]. When activated, PHDs enhance hydroxylation of specific prolyl and asparagyl residues of the transcription protein, hypoxia-inducible factor 1 (HIF-1). HIF-1 is composed of two subunits, HIF-1α and HIF-1β. HIF-1β is constitutively expressed whereas HIF-1α protein is highly unstable, and its accumulation is regulated by the von Hippel–Lindau (VHL) protein, an E3-ubiquitin ligase. Under normoxic condition, this ligase targets HIF-1α to the proteasomal degradation. Conversely, in hypoxic conditions, HIF-1α is not recognized by VHL. It translocates to the nucleus and forms a complex with HIF1-β, which binds to a HIF response element present in HIF target genes. HIF-1α negatively regulates chondrocytes proliferation and promotes their survival [118, 141].

Apoptosis: Apoptosis of hypertrophic chondrocyte, which occurs at the cartilage vascular interface, is central to endochondral ossification and elongation. Changes in mitochondrial function initiated by early apoptotic events and modulated by the Bcl-2 (B-cell leukemia/lymphoma 2) family of proteins regulate calcium accumulation and release [107, 109]. Calcium released from hypertrophic chondrocytes generates matrix calcification nucleated by matrix vesicles, the remnants of apoptotic chondrocytes. Apoptosis triggered events lead to activation of pretenses on the cell surface and within the matrix, and the destruction of the cartilage matrix. Apoptosis initiated activation and release of growth factors regulates the homeostatic maintenance of growth plate width, stimulation of blood vessel invasion, stimulation of osteoblast recruitment, and the formation of blood vessels and osteoid [142]. Chondrocyte apoptosis is regulated by signals triggered by local factors such as FGF-2 that leads to increased apoptosis or PTHrP that upregulates Bcl-2 expression as part of its mechanism to control the rate of chondrocyte turnover [107].

2.6   Osteoclast

Bone fracture is followed by a unique healing process, which initially shares certain features with healing processes in other connective tissues. The injury may involve consequent to the location, cortical bone, periosteum, bone marrow and additional soft tissues. The trauma sets off an inflammatory response characterized by a series of molecular and cellular events concurrent with substantial MSC recruitment.

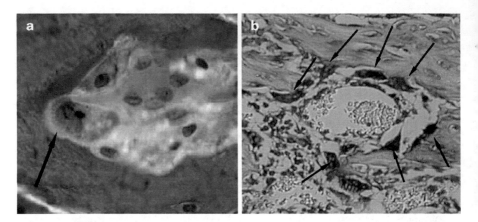

Fig. 2.10 Histological features of osteoclasts. (**a**) A typical appearance of osteoclasts in bone remodelling unit (*arrow*) in H&E Stain. (**b**) Osteoclasts (*arrows*) in tartarate-resistant acid phosphatase staining (*red*)

This is followed by the emergence of a large number of osteoclasts, primarily responsible for an extensive cartilage and bone resorption, in which the mineralized constituent and the organic matrix are disintegrated (Fig. 2.10). Concomitantly, endothelial cells initiate angiogenesis and progenitor cells differentiate into chondroblasts and osteoblasts that form a bridging callus at the fracture gap. Further resorption and ossification brings about restoration of the original bone. Callus remodeling concludes with the regeneration of a mechanically competent osseous structure.

Origin and Genesis of Osteoclasts. The osteoclast is a multinuclear phagocyte derived from bone marrow HSCs. These cells serve as a common origin to all blood cells as well as other members of the immune system. Multinucleation is ascribed to the fusion of precursor monocytes. The osteoclast constitutes an essential linkage between the immune and the osseous systems. Evidently, a variety of cytokines, their receptors, and downstream signaling pathways are operative in both systems. Cells of the osteoblastic lineage, as well as immune cells, express factors that induce osteoclast formation. Among those, macrophage colony stimulating factor (M-CSF), receptor–activator of NFκB ligand (RANKL), and tumor necrosis factor (TNF) are counted. These factors induce mononuclear cells to fuse and form multinucleated osteoclasts with bone-resorbing capability. Such factors are minimally expressed in intact bone. However, they are markedly increased following bone fracture [143, 144]. These factors, in particular M-CSF and RANKL, are essential for osteoclastogenesis. Their expression is markedly increased before the onset of calcified cartilage removal. Fracture healing in mice deficient of these cytokines is prolonged due to blockade of the transition of calcified cartilage to bone. Such deficiencies could be involved in the etiology of a subclass of nonunion fractures, which demonstrate the persistence of calcified cartilaginous callus [145]. Cellular multinucleation is the key feature distinguishing osteoclasts from their precursors. Dendritic cell-specific

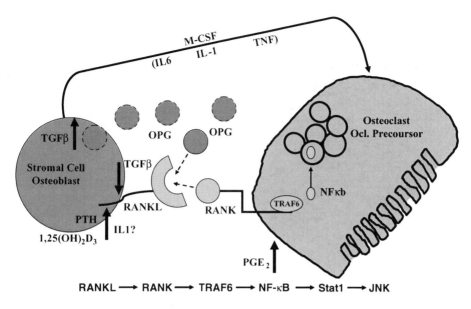

Fig. 2.11   Stromal cell–osteoclast interaction

transmembrane protein (DC-STAMP) was found to be critical for fusion of the mononuclear precursors to form multinucleated osteoclasts. DC-STAMP-deficient cells fail to fuse, yet exhibit normal features of an osteoclast with actin ring and ruffled border formation [146]. The current hypothesis regarding the developmental stages from the firstly identifiable osteoclast precursor to the mature active resorbing cells is illustrated in Fig. 2.11.

The M-CSF-RANKL system has been in the focus of osteoclast research for more than a decade. In the presence of M-CSF RANKL activated its receptor, RANK, leading monocytes/macrophages into the osteoclastic pathway [147]. RANKL is mostly a membrane anchored protein of the osteoblast lineage. Hence, a cell–cell interaction is required for its action. However, this may not be the whole scenario, as soluble RANKL is produced by T cells and is osteoclastogenic, together with M-CSF, ex vivo cultures. The divergence from the macrophage/dendritic cell toward the osteoclast is shown in Fig. 2.10b. An important modifier of the RANKL–RANK interaction is system OPG, produced by several cells and tissues including osteoblasts and stromal cells. Like RANK, OPG belongs to the TNF receptor family and acts as a soluble decoy receptor, competing with RANK on the binding to RANKL, thus inhibiting osteoclastogenesis [148, 149].

Migration and Targeting. Conceptually, bone resorption should involve the recruitment of osteoclasts and/or their precursors to the site of degradation of the mineralized matrix. Indeed, several matrix proteins such as type I collagen peptides, a2HS glycoprotein, osteocalcin, and stromal cell-derived factor-1 demonstrate monocyte chemoattraction. Whether they function in this capacity remains to be investigated.

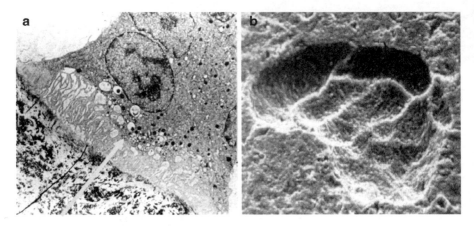

Fig. 2.12 Osteoclastic resorption. (**a**) Transmission electron micrograph of an actively resorbing osteoclast. Note, Ruffled border (*arrow*). (**b**) Howship's Lacunae/*ex vivo* pit formation

Another class of chemotactic signals could originate in osteocytes. The association between micro cracks to bone remodeling raised the suggestion that dying osteocytes at the crack site may signal to the attraction of osteoclast precursors [150]. Also, intact osteocytes may inhibit resorption; when the osteocyte originating osteoclast restraining signals are alleviated, the osteoclast precursors could migrate toward the fracture site [151]. Matrix metalloproteinases (MMPs) were found to be critical for the migration of the precursor cells. MMP14 in particular carves the path for osteoclastic cell migration through the degradation of non-mineralized matrices. In addition, MMP9 could probably release chemo-attractants like vascular endothelial growth factor (VEGF) [152].

2.6.1 Structure and Function

The osteoclast is a large (~300 mm) cell with up to eight nuclei. The reason for these features is unclear. The osteoclast has two major opposite plasma membrane domains, the functional secretory domain (FSD) that faces the mineralized matrix and the basolateral domain (BLD), usually in a close proximity to a blood vessel [147, 153]. At the FSD the cytoskeleton reorganizes and assumes polarization of F-actin to a circular structure, the "actin ring." The plasma membrane beneath the actin ring forms a tight attachment with the mineralized matrix. The attachment mediated by avb3 integrin through the recognition of bone protein sequences such as osteopontin and sialoprotein. The primary adhesion structures of osteoclasts are dot-like, actin-rich structures known as podosomes. This attachment outlines the sealed zone, which is the space between the mineralized matrix and a highly convoluted, ruffled, resorbing part of the osteoclast cell membrane (Fig. 2.12). Hydrogen ions and matrix degrading enzymes are secreted into the sealed zone through the ruffled

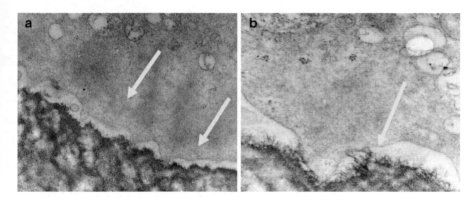

Fig. 2.13 Transmission electron micrographs of seal zone. Note, Podosomes (*arrows*)

membrane. Mineral dissolution and organic matrix degradation are followed by removal of the products from the resorption lacuna. This step involves transcytosis and secretion into the circulation at the BLD [154].

Mineral Dissolution and Organic Component Degradation. Osteoclast attachment to bone with isolation of a sealed space and formation of a ruffled border (Fig. 2.13) creates a secluded compartment at the resorption site. Acidified conditions of pH ~4.5 develop at this location by the generation of hydrochloric acid (HCl) that dissolved the bone mineral. The HCl is formed by the mobilization of hydrogen (H^+) and chlorine (Cl^-) ions from inside the osteoclast across the ruffled membrane. The HCl is mobilized by fusion of acidic vesicles with the ruffled border coupled to an electrogenic proton pump (H^+-ATPase) coupled with a Cl^- channel. The functional separation of the ruffled border from the rest of the cell membrane by the sealing zone enables concentration of the HCl. To enable a constant release of HCl into the resorption area, protons are continuously produced by the activity of carbonic anhydrase II, an enzyme that is highly expressed in osteoclasts and facilitates the hydration of CO_2, resulting in the production of protons and HCO_3^-. The latter is substituted to chloride by the chloride-bicarbonate exchanger located in the basolateral membrane. The osteoclast is characterized also by a high number of mitochondria required to produce energy for the resorption process. The organic matrix is degraded probably by more than one enzyme. It seems, however, that cathepsin K is the main bone matrix breakdown enzyme [155] (Fig. 2.14).

Osteoclastic Bone Resorption. Carbonic anhydrase II catalyzes the hydration of CO_2 resulting in the supply of protons that accumulate in the resorption area by proton pump and through vesicular transport (Fig. 2.14). The HCO_3^- produced together with the proton is exchanged for chloride ions that are transferred through chloride channels into the resorption area. The HCl dissolves the hydroxyapatite and cathepsin K exocytosed from the cell degrades the collagen. The ions and collagen degradation products are endocytosed by the ruffled membrane, the vesicles

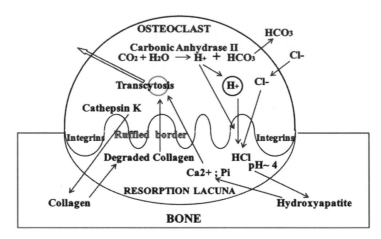

Fig. 2.14 Osteoclastic bone resorption

are fused to the membrane opposite to the ruffled membranes, and the resorption products are disposed.

Disposal of Resorption Products. Efficient resorption requires an instantaneous removal of the ions and the collagen fragments produced. The FSD is the area where degradation products are targeted [156]. They are endocytosed into the osteoclast. The endocytic vesicles, derived from the ruffled border, fuse with the FSD, and the degradation products are released into the extracellular fluid, mainly the blood stream, at the BLD.

Mineralized Tissue Resorption in Bone Healing. Osteoclasts have a key role in the cartilage-to-bone transition of fracture healing and in the consequent remodeling and maturation of the bony callus toward regeneration of the cortical bone. It has been shown that inhibition of bone resorption during fracture healing, by agents such as bisphosphonates, leads to enlarged callus and delays its replacement by bone. The biomechanical properties of the consequential bony callus are diminished [157]. Increased resorption, as in the case of partially stabilized and fractures and bone injuries in aged individuals, is associated with diminished trabecular bone parameters and callus strength [158]. Although the clinical significance of these findings has not been fully elaborated, special care, such as rigid fixation, and a close follow-up should be implemented in elderly patients and those receiving anti-resorptive medication.

References

1. Gordeladze JO, Djouad F, Brondello JM, Noël D, Duroux-Richard I, Apparailly F, Jorgensen C (2009) Concerted stimuli regulating osteo-chondral differentiation from stem cells: phenotype acquisition regulated by microRNAs. Acta Pharmacol Sin 30:1369–1384

2. Ahdjoudj S, Fromigué O, Marie PJ (2004) Plasticity and regulation of human bone marrow stromal osteoprogenitor cells: potential implication in the treatment of age-related bone loss. Histol Histopathol 19:151–157
3. Qi H, Aguiar DJ, Williams SM, La Pean A, Pan W, Verfaillie CM (2003) Identification of genes responsible for osteoblast differentiation from human mesodermal progenitor cells. Proc Natl Acad Sci USA 100:3305–3310
4. Jensen ED, Gopalakrishnan R, Westendorf JJ (2010) Regulation of Gene Expression in Osteoblasts. Biofactors 36:25
5. Gabet Y, Muller R, Regev E, Sela J, Shteyer A, Salisbury K, Chorev M, Bab I (2004) Osteogenic growth peptide modulates fracture callus structural and mechanical properties. Bone 35:65–73
6. Muruganandan S, Roman A, Sinal CJ (2009) Role of chemerin/CMKLR1 signaling in adipogenesis and osteoblastogenesis of bone marrow stem cells. J Bone Miner Res 25:222–234
7. Muruganandan S, Roman AA, Sinal CJ (2009) Adipocyte differentiation of bone marrow-derived mesenchymal stem cells: cross talk with the osteoblastogenic program. Cell Mol Life Sci 66:236–253, Review
8. Tapscott SJ (2005) The circuitry of a master switch: Myod and the regulation of skeletal muscle gene transcription. Development 132:2685–2695
9. Tontonoz P, Spiegelman BM (2008) Fat and beyond: the diverse biology of PPARgamma. Annu Rev Biochem 77:289–312
10. de Crombrugghe B, Lefebvre V, Behringer RR, Bi W, Murakami S, Huang W (2000) Transcriptional mechanisms of chondrocyte differentiation. Matrix Biol 19:389–394
11. Otto F, Thornell AP, Crompton T, Denzel A, Gilmour KC, Rosewell IR, Stamp GW, Beddington RS, Mundlos S, Olsen BR, Selby PB, Owen MJ (1997) Cbfa1, a candidate gene for cleidocranial dysplasia syndrome, is essential for osteoblast differentiation and bone development. Cell 89:765–771
12. Shalhoub V, Gerstenfeld LC, Collart D, Lian JB, Stein GS (1989) Downregulation of cell growth and cell cycle regulated genes during chick osteoblast differentiation with the reciprocal expression of histone gene variants. Biochemistry 28:5318–5322
13. Stein GS, Lian JB, Gerstenfeld LG, Shalhoub V, Aronow M, Owen T, Markose E (1989) The onset and progression of osteoblast differentiation is functionally related to cellular proliferation. Connect Tissue Res 20:3–13
14. Stein GS, Lian JB, van Wijnen AJ, Stein JL, Montecino M, Javed A, Zaidi SK, Young DW, Choi JY, Pockwinse SM (2004) Runx2 control of organization, assembly and activity of the regulatory machinery for skeletal gene expression. Oncogene 23:4315–4329
15. Mundlos S, Otto F, Mundlos C, Mulliken JB, Aylsworth AS, Albright S, Lindhout D, Cole WG, Henn W, Knoll JH, Owen MJ, Mertelsmann R, Zabel BU, Olsen BR (1997) Mutations involving the transcription factor CBFA1 cause cleidocranial dysplasia. Cell 89:773–779
16. Jensen ED, Nair AK, Westendorf JJ (2007) Histone deacetylase co-repressor complex control of Runx2 and bone formation. Crit Rev Eukaryot Gene Expr 17:187–196
17. Schroeder TM, Jensen ED, Westendorf JJ (2005) Runx2: a master organizer of gene transcription in developing and maturing osteoblasts. Birth Defects Res C Embryo Today 75:213–225
18. Komori T, Yagi H, Nomura S, Yamaguchi A, Sasaki K, Deguchi K, Shimizu Y, Bronson RT, Gao YH, Inada M, Sato M, Okamoto R, Kitamura Y, Yoshiki S, Kishimoto T (1997) Targeted disruption of Cbfa1 results in a complete lack of bone formation owing to maturational arrest of osteoblasts. Cell 89:755–764
19. Pelletier N, Champagne N, Stifani S, Yang XJ (2002) MOZ and MORF histone acetyltransferases interact with the Runt-domain transcription factor Runx2. Oncogene 21:2729–2740
20. Sierra J, Villagra A, Paredes R, Cruzat F, Gutierrez S, Javed A, Arriagada G, Olate J, Imschenetzky M, Van Wijnen AJ, Lian JB, Stein GS, Stein JL, Montecino M (2003) Regulation of the bone-specific osteocalcin gene by p300 requires Runx2/Cbfa1 and the vitamin D3 receptor but not p300 intrinsic histone acetyltransferase activity. Mol Cell Biol 23:3339–3351
21. Westendorf JJ, Zaidi SK, Cascino JE, Kahler R, van Wijnen AJ, Lian JB, Yoshida M, Stein GS, Li X (2002) Runx2 (Cbfa1, AML-3) interacts with histone deacetylase 6 and represses the p21 (CIP1/WAF1) promoter. Mol Cell Biol 22:7982–7992

22. Jensen ED, Schroeder TM, Bailey J, Gopalakrishnan R, Westendorf JJ (2008) Histone deacetylase 7 associates with Runx2 and represses its activity during osteoblast maturation in a deacetylation-independent manner. J Bone Miner Res 23:361–372

23. Jeon EJ, Lee KY, Choi NS, Lee MH, Kim HN, Jin YH, Ryoo HM, Choi JY, Yoshida M, Nishino N, Oh BC, Lee KS, Lee YH, Bae SC (2006) Bone morphogenetic protein-2 stimulates Runx2 acetylation. J Biol Chem 281:16502–16511

24. Schroeder TM, Kahler RA, Li X, Westendorf JJ (2004) Histone deacetylase 3 interacts with runx2 to repress the osteocalcin promoter and regulate osteoblast differentiation. J Biol Chem 279:41998–42007

25. Vega RB, Matsuda K, Oh J, Barbosa AC, Yang X, Meadows E, McAnally J, Pomajzl C, Shelton JM, Richardson JA, Karsenty G, Olson EN (2004) Histone deacetylase 4 controls chondrocyte hypertrophy during skeletogenesis. Cell 119:555–566

26. Choo MK, Yeo H, Zayzafoon M (2009) NFATc1 mediates HDAC-dependent transcriptional repression of osteocalcin expression during osteoblast differentiation. Bone 45:579–589

27. Lamour V, Detry C, Sanchez C, Henrotin Y, Castronovo V, Bellahcene A (2007) Runx2- and histone deacetylase 3-mediated repression is relieved in differentiating human osteoblast cells to allow high bone sialoprotein expression. J Biol Chem 282:36240–36249

28. Schroeder TM, Westendorf JJ (2005) Histone deacetylase inhibitors promote osteoblast maturation. J Bone Miner Res 20:2254–2263

29. Cho HH, Park HT, Kim YJ, Bae YC, Suh KT, Jung JS (2005) Induction of osteogenic differentiation of human mesenchymal stem cells by histone deacetylase inhibitors. J Cell Biochem 96:533–542

30. Lee HW, Suh JH, Kim AY, Lee YS, Park SY, Kim JB (2006) Histone deacetylase 1-mediated histone modification regulates osteoblast differentiation. Mol Endocrinol 20:2432–2443

31. Tintut Y, Parhami F, Le V, Karsenty G, Demer LL (1999) Inhibition of osteoblast-specific transcription factor Cbfa1 by the cAMP pathway in osteoblastic cells. Ubiquitin/proteasome-dependent regulation. J Biol Chem 274:28875–28879

32. Zhao M, Qiao M, Oyajobi BO, Mundy GR, Chen D (2003) E3 ubiquitin ligase Smurf1 mediates core-binding factor alpha1/Runx2 degradation and plays a specific role in osteoblast differentiation. J Biol Chem 278:27939–27944

33. Jones DC, Wein MN, Glimcher LH (2007) Schnurri-3: a key regulator of postnatal skeletal remodeling. Adv Exp Med Biol 602:1–13

34. Jones DC, Wein MN, Oukka M, Hofstaetter JG, Glimcher MJ, Glimcher LH (2006) Regulation of adult bone mass by the zinc finger adapter protein Schnurri-3. Science 312:1223–1227

35. Glimcher LH, Jones DC, Wein MN (2007) Control of postnatal bone mass by the zinc finger adapter protein Schnurri-3. Ann N Y Acad Sci 1116:174–181

36. Bellido T, Ali AA, Plotkin LI, Fu Q, Gubrij I, Roberson PK, Weinstein RS, O'Brien CA, Manolagas SC, Jilka RL (2003) Proteasomal degradation of Runx2 shortens parathyroid hormone-induced anti-apoptotic signaling in osteoblasts. A putative explanation for why intermittent administration is needed for bone anabolism. J Biol Chem 278:50259–50272

37. Jeong BC, Lee YS, Park YY, Bae IH, Kim DK, Koo SH, Choi HR, Kim SH, Franceschi RT, Koh JT, Choi HS (2009) The orphan nuclear receptor estrogen receptor-related receptor gamma negatively regulates BMP2-induced osteoblast differentiation and bone formation. J Biol Chem 284:14211–14218

38. Jensen ED, Gopalakrishnan R, Westendorf JJ (2009) Bone morphogenic protein 2 activates protein kinase D to regulate histone deacetylase 7 localization and repression of Runx2. J Biol Chem 284:2225–2234

39. Porte D, Tuckermann J, Becker M, Baumann B, Teurich S, Higgins T, Owen MJ, Schorpp-Kistner M, Angel P (1999) Both AP-1 and Cbfa1-like factors are required for the induction of interstitial collagenase by parathyroid hormone. Oncogene 18:667–678

40. Winchester SK, Selvamurugan N, D'Alonzo RC, Partridge NC (2000) Developmental regulation of collagenase-3 mRNA in normal, differentiating osteoblasts through the activator protein-1 and the runt domain binding sites. J Biol Chem 275:23310–23318

41. Boumah CE, Lee M, Selvamurugan N, Shimizu E, Partridge NC (2009) Runx2 recruits p300 to mediate parathyroid hormone's effects on histone acetylation and transcriptional activation of the matrix metalloproteinase-13 gene. Mol Endocrinol 23:1255–1263
42. Selvamurugan N, Pulumati MR, Tyson DR, Partridge NC (2000) Parathyroid hormone regulation of the rat collagenase-3 promoter by protein kinase A-dependent transactivation of core binding factor alpha1. J Biol Chem 275:5037–5042
43. D'Alonzo RC, Selvamurugan N, Karsenty G, Partridge NC (2002) Physical interaction of the activator protein-1 factors c-Fos and c-Jun with Cbfa1 for collagenase-3 promoter activation. J Biol Chem 277:816–822
44. Selvamurugan N, Jefcoat SC, Kwok S, Kowalewski R, Tamasi JA, Partridge NC (2006) Overexpression of Runx2 directed by the matrix metalloproteinase-13 promoter containing the AP-1 and Runx/RD/Cbfa sites alters bone remodeling in vivo. J Cell Biochem 99:545–557
45. Nakashima K, Zhou X, Kunkel G, Zhang Z, Deng JM, Behringer RR, de Crombrugghe B (2002) The novel zinc finger-containing transcription factor osterix is required for osteoblast differentiation and bone formation. Cell 108:17–29
46. Nishio Y, Dong Y, Paris M, O'Keefe RJ, Schwarz EM, Drissi H (2006) Runx2-mediated regulation of zinc finger Osterix/Sp7 gene. Gene 372:62–70
47. Koga T, Matsui Y, Asagiri M, Kodama T, de Crombrugghe B, Nakashima K, Takayanagi H (2005) NFAT and Osterix cooperatively regulate bone formation. Nat Med 11:880–885
48. Zhang C, Cho K, Huang Y, Lyons JP, Zhou X, Sinha K, McCrea PD, de Crombrugghe B (2008) Inhibition of Wnt signaling by the osteoblast-specific transcription factor Osterix. Proc Natl Acad Sci USA 105:6936–6941
49. Yang X, Matsuda K, Bialek P, Jacquot S, Masuoka HC, Schinke T, Li L, Brancorsini S, Sassone-Corsi P, Townes TM, Hanauer A, Karsenty G (2004) ATF4 is a substrate of RSK2 and an essential regulator of osteoblast biology; implication for Coffin-Lowry Synd. Cell 117:387–398
50. Yang X, Karsenty G (2004) ATF4, the osteoblast accumulation of which is determined post-translationally, can induce osteoblast-specific gene expression in non-osteoblastic cells. J Biol Chem 279:47109–47114
51. Xiao G, Jiang D, Ge C, Zhao Z, Lai Y, Boules H, Phimphilai M, Yang X, Karsenty G, Franceschi RT (2005) Cooperative interactions between activating transcription factor 4 and Runx2/Cbfa1 stimulate osteoblast-specific osteocalcin gene expression. J Biol Chem 280:30689–30696
52. Yu S, Franceschi RT, Luo M, Zhang X, Jiang D, Lai Y, Jiang Y, Zhang J, Xiao G (2008) Parathyroid hormone increases activating transcription factor 4 expression and activity in osteoblasts: requirement for osteocalcin gene expression. Endocrinology 149:1960–1968
53. Tominaga H, Maeda S, Hayashi M, Takeda S, Akira S, Komiya S, Nakamura T, Akiyama H, Imamura T (2008) CCAAT/enhancer-binding protein beta promotes osteoblast differentiation by enhancing Runx2 activity with ATF4. Mol Biol Cell 19:5373–5386
54. Yu S, Jiang Y, Galson DL, Luo M, Lai Y, Lu Y, Ouyang HJ, Zhang J, Xiao G (2008) General transcription factor IIA-gamma increases osteoblast-specific osteocalcin gene expression via activating transcription factor 4 and runt-related transcription factor 2. J Biol Chem 283:5542–5553
55. Hinoi E, Gao N, Jung DY, Yadav V, Yoshizawa T, Kajimura D, Myers MG Jr, Chua SC Jr, Wang Q, Kim JK, Kaestner KH, Karsenty G (2009) An osteoblast-dependent mechanism contributes to the leptin regulation of insulin secretion. Ann N Y Acad Sci 1173(Suppl 1):E20–E30
56. Yoshizawa T, Hinoi E, Jung DY, Kajimura D, Ferron M, Seo J, Graff JM, Kim JK, Karsenty G (2009) The transcription factor ATF4 regulates glucose metabolism in mice through its expression in osteoblasts. J Clin Invest 119:2807–2817
57. Lee KS, Kim HJ, Li QL, Chi XZ, Ueta C, Komori T, Wozney JM, Kim EG, Choi JY, Ryoo HM, Bae SC (2000) Runx2 is a common target of transforming growth factor beta1 and bone morphogenetic protein 2, and cooperation between Runx2 and Smad5 induces osteoblast-specific gene expression in the pluripotent mesenchymal precursor cell line C2C12. Mol Cell Biol 20:8783–8792

58. Bae JS, Gutierrez S, Narla R, Pratap J, Devados R, van Wijnen AJ, Stein JL, Stein GS, Lian JB, Javed A (2007) Reconstitution of Runx2/Cbfa1-null cells identifies a requirement for BMP2 signaling through a Runx2 functional domain during osteoblast differentiation. J Cell Biochem 100:434–449

59. Hanai J, Chen LF, Kanno T, Ohtani-Fujita N, Kim WY, Guo WH, Imamura T, Ishidou Y, Fukuchi M, Shi MJ, Stavnezer J, Kawabata M, Miyazono K, Ito Y (1999) Interaction and functional cooperation of PEBP2/CBF with Smads. Synergistic induction of the immunoglobulin germline Calpha promoter. J Biol Chem 274:31577–31582

60. Javed A, Afzal F, Bae JS, Gutierrez S, Zaidi K, Pratap J, van Wijnen AJ, Stein JL, Stein GS, Lian JB (2009) Specific residues of RUNX2 are obligatory for formation of BMP2-induced RUNX2-SMAD complex to promote osteoblast differentiation. Cells Tissues Organs 189:133–137

61. Javed A, Bae JS, Afzal F, Gutierrez S, Pratap J, Zaidi SK, Lou Y, van Wijnen AJ, Stein JL, Stein GS, Lian JB (2008) Structural coupling of Smad and Runx2 for execution of the BMP2 osteogenic signal. J Biol Chem 283:8412–8422

62. Afzal F, Pratap J, Ito K, Ito Y, Stein JL, van Wijnen AJ, Stein GS, Lian JB, Javed A (2005) Smad function and intranuclear targeting share a Runx2 motif required for osteogenic lineage induction and BMP2 responsive transcription. J Cell Physiol 204:63–72

63. Wang Q, Wei X, Zhu T, Zhang M, Shen R, Xing L, O'Keefe RJ, Chen D (2007) Bone morphogenetic protein 2 activates Smad6 gene transcription through bone-specific transcription factor Runx2. J Biol Chem 282:10742–10748

64. Shen R, Chen M, Wang YJ, Kaneki H, Xing L, O'Keefe JR, Chen D (2006) Smad6 interacts with Runx2 and mediates Smad ubiquitin regulatory factor 1-induced Runx2 degradation. J Biol Chem 281:3569–3576

65. Hogan PG, Chen L, Nardone J, Rao A (2003) Transcriptional regulation by calcium, calcineurin, and NFAT. Genes Dev 17:2205–2232

66. Bourgeois P, Bolcato-Bellemin AL, Danse JM, Bloch-Zupan A, Yoshiba K, Stoetzel C, Perrin-Schmitt F (1998) The variable expressivity and incomplete penetrance of the twist-null heterozygous mouse phenotype resemble those of human Saethre-Chotzen syndrome. Hum Mol Genet 7:945–957

67. el Ghouzzi V, Le Merrer M, Perrin-Schmitt F, Lajeunie E, Benit P, Renier D, Bourgeois P, Bolcato-Bellemin AL, Munnich A, Bonaventure J (1997) Mutations of the TWIST gene in the Saethre-Chotzen syndrome. Nat Genet 15:42–46

68. Howard TD, Paznekas WA, Green ED, Chiang LC, Ma N, Ortiz de Luna RI, Garcia Delgado C, Gonzalez-Ramos M, Kline AD, Jabs EW (1997) Mutations in TWIST, a basic helix-loop-helix transcription factor, in Saethre-Chotzen syndrome. Nat Genet 15:36–41

69. Bialek P, Kern B, Yang X, Schrock M, Sosic D, Hong N, Wu H, Yu K, Ornitz DM, Olson EN, Justice MJ, Karsenty G (2004) A twist code determines onset of osteoblast differentiation. Dev Cell 6:423–435

70. Hayashi M, Nimura K, Kashiwagi K, Harada T, Takaoka K, Kato H, Tamai K, Kaneda Y (2007) Comparative roles of Twist-1& Id1in transcriptional regulation by BMP signaling. J Cell Sci 120:1350–1357

71. McCabe LR, Banerjee C, Kundu R, Harrison RJ, Dobner PR, Stein JL, Lian JB, Stein GS (1996) Developmental expression and activities of specific Fos and jun proteins are functionally related to osteoblast maturation: role of Fra-2 and Jun D during differentiation. Endocrinology 137:4398–4408

72. Grigoriadis AE, Wang ZQ, Cecchini MG, Hofstetter W, Felix R, Fleisch HA, Wagner EF (1994) c-Fos: a key regulator of osteoclast-macrophage lineage determination and bone remodeling. Science 266:443–448

73. Grigoriadis AE, Schellander K, Wang ZQ, Wagner EF (1993) Osteoblasts are target cells for transformation in c-fos transgenic mice. J Cell Biol 122:685–701

74. Jochum W, David JP, Elliott C, Wutz A, Plenk H Jr, Matsuo K, Wagner EF (2000) Increased bone formation and osteosclerosis in mice overexpressing the transcription factor Fra-1. Nat Med 6:980–984

75. Sabatakos G, Sims NA, Chen J, Aoki K, Kelz MB, Amling M, Bouali Y, Mukhopadhyay K, Ford K, Nestler EJ, Baron R (2000) Overexpression of DeltaFosB transcription factor (s) increases bone formation and inhibits adipogenesis. Nat Med 6:985–990

76. Chang J, Wang Z, Tang E, Fan Z, McCauley L, Franceschi R, Guan K, Krebsbach PH, Wang CY (2009) Inhibition of osteoblastic bone formation by nuclear factor-kappa B. Nat Med 15:682–689

77. Owen TA, Bortell R, Yocum SA, Smock SL, Zhang M, Abate C, Shalhoub V, Aronin N, Wright KL, van Wijnen AJ et al (1990) Coordinate occupancy of AP-1 sites in the vitamin D-responsive and CCAAT box elements by Fos-Jun in the osteocalcin gene: model for phenotype suppression of transcription. Proc Natl Acad Sci USA 87:9990–9994

78. Sabatakos G, Rowe GC, Kveiborg M, Wu M, Neff L, Chiusaroli R, Philbrick WM, Baron R (2008) Doubly truncated FosB isoform (Delta2DeltaFosB) induces osteosclerosis in transgenic mice and modulates expression and phosphorylation of Smads in osteoblasts independent of intrinsic AP-1 activity. J Bone Miner Res 23:584–595

79. Behrens J, von Kries JP, Kuhl M, Bruhn L, Wedlich D, Grosschedl R, Birchmeier W (1996) Functional interaction of beta-catenin with the transcription factor LEF-1. Nature 382:638–642

80. Billin AN, Thirlwell H, Ayer DE (2000) Beta-catenin-histone deacetylase interactions regulate the transition of LEF1 from a transcriptional repressor to an activator. Mol Cell Biol 20:6882–6890

81. Chen G, Fernandez J, Mische S, Courey AJ (1999) A functional interaction between the histone deacetylase Rpd3 and the corepressor groucho in Drosophila development. Genes Dev 13:2218–2230

82. Daniels DL, Weis WI (2005) Beta-catenin directly displaces Groucho/TLE repressors from Tcf/Lef in Wnt-mediated transcription activation. Nat Struct Mol Biol 12:364–371

83. Hecht A, Vleminckx K, Stemmler MP, van Roy F, Kemler R (2000) The p300/CBP acetyltransferases function as transcriptional coactivators of beta-catenin in vertebrates. EMBO J 19:1839–1850

84. Glass DA 2nd, Bialck P, Ahn JD, Starbuck M, Patel MS, Clevers H, Taketo MM, Long F, McMahon AP, Lang RA, Karsenty G (2005) Canonical wnt signaling in differentiated osteoblasts controls osteoclast differentiation. Dev Cell 8:751–764

85. Kahler RA, Westendorf JJ (2003) Lymphoid enhancer factor-1 and beta-catenin inhibit Runx2-dependent transcriptional activation of the osteocalcin promoter. J Biol Chem 278:11937–11944

86. Oosterwegel M, van de Wetering M, Timmerman J, Kruisbeek A, Destree O, Meijlink F, Clevers H (1993) Differential expression of the HMG box factors TCF-1 and LEF-1 during murine embryogenesis. Development 118:439–448

87. van Genderen C, Okamura RM, Farinas I, Quo RG, Parslow TG, Bruhn L, Grosschedl R (1994) Development of several organs that require inductive epithelial-mesenchymal interactions is impaired in LEF-1-deficient mice. Genes Dev 8:2691–2703

88. Noh T, Gabet Y, Cogan J, Shi Y, Tank A, Sasaki T, Criswell B, Dixon A, Lee C, Tam J, Kohler T, Segev E, Kockeritz L, Woodgett J, Muller R, Chai Y, Smith E, Bab I, Frenkel B (2009) Lef1 haploinsufficient mice display a low turnover and low bone mass phenotype in a gender- and age-specific manner. PLoS One 4:e5438

89. Kahler RA, Galindo M, Lian J, Stein GS, van Wijnen AJ, Westendorf JJ (2006) Lymphocyte enhancer-binding factor 1 (Lef1) inhibits terminal differentiation of osteoblasts. J Cell Biochem 97:969–983

90. Hoeppner LH, Secreto F, Jensen ED, Li X, Kahler RA, Westendorf JJ (2009) Runx2 and bone morphogenic protein 2 regulate the expression of an alternative Lef1 transcript during osteoblast maturation. J Cell Physiol 221:480–489

91. Gaur T, Lengner CJ, Hovhannisyan H, Bhat RA, Bodine PV, Komm BS, Javed A, van Wijnen AJ, Stein JL, Stein GS, Lian JB (2005) Canonical WNT signaling promotes osteogenesis by directly stimulating Runx2 gene expression. J Biol Chem 280:33132–33140

92. Bain G, Muller T, Wang X, Papkoff J (2003) Activated beta-catenin induces osteoblast differentiation of C3H10T1/2 cells and participates in BMP2 mediated signal transduction. Biochem Biophys Res Commun 301:84–91

93. Qiang YW, Barlogie B, Rudikoff S, Shaughnessy JD (2008) Jr Dkk1-induced inhibition of Wnt signaling in osteoblast differentiation is an underlying mechanism of bone loss in multiple myeloma. Bone 42:669–680

94. Rawadi G, Vayssiere B, Dunn F, Baron R, Roman-Roman S (2003) BMP-2 controls alkaline phosphatase expression and osteoblast mineralization by a Wnt autocrine loop. J Bone Miner Res 18:1842–1853

95. Ambrosetti D, Holmes G, Mansukhani A, Basilico C (2008) Fibroblast growth factor signaling uses multiple mechanisms to inhibit Wnt-induced transcription in osteoblasts. Mol Cell Biol 28:4759–4771

96. Wu M, Hesse E, Morvan F, Zhang JP, Correa D, Rowe GC, Kiviranta R, Neff L, Philbrick WM, Horne WC, Baron R (2009) Zfp521 antagonizes Runx2, delays osteoblast differentiation in vitro, and promotes bone formation in vivo. Bone 44:528–536

97. Zhang Y, Hassan MQ, Xie RL, Hawse JR, Spelsberg TC, Montecino M, Stein JL, Lian JB, van Wijnen AJ, Stein GS (2009) Co-stimulation of the bone-related Runx2 P1 promoter in mesenchymal cells by SP1 and ETS transcription factors at polymorphic purine-rich DNA sequences (Y-repeats). J Biol Chem 284:3125–3135

98. Lai CF, Feng X, Nishimura R, Teitelbaum SL, Avioli LV, Ross FP, Cheng SL (2000) Transforming growth factor-beta up-regulates the beta 5 integrin subunit expression via Sp1 and Smad signaling. J Biol Chem 275:36400–36406

99. Suttamanatwong S, Jensen ED, Schilling J, Franceschi RT, Carlson AE, Mansky KC, Gopalakrishnan R (2009) Sp proteins and Runx2 mediate regulation of matrix gla protein (MGP) expression by parathyroid hormone. J Cell Biochem 107:284–292

100. Erson AE, Petty EM (2008) MicroRNAs in development and disease. Clin Genet 74:296–306

101. Li Z, Hassan MQ, Volinia S, van Wijnen AJ, Stein JL, Croce CM, Lian JB, Stein GS (2008) A microRNA signature for a BMP2-induced osteoblast lineage commitment program. Proc Natl Acad Sci USA 105:13906–13911

102. Itoh T, Nozawa Y, Akao Y (2009) MicroRNA-141 and -200a are involved in bone morphogenetic protein-2-induced mouse pre-osteoblast differentiation by targeting distal-less homeobox 5. J Biol Chem 284:19272–19279

103. Kapinas K, Kessler CB, Delany AM (2009) miR-29 suppression of osteonectin in osteoblasts: regulation during differentiation and by canonical Wnt signaling. J Cell Biochem 108:216–224

104. Mizuno Y, Tokuzawa Y, Ninomiya Y, Yagi K, Yatsuka-Kanesaki Y, Suda T, Fukuda T, Katagiri T, Kondoh Y, Amemiya T, Tashiro H, Okazaki Y (2009) miR-210 promotes osteoblastic differentiation through inhibition of AcvR1b. FEBS Lett 583:2263–2268

105. Nilsson O, Marino R, De Luca F, Phillip M, Baron J (2005) Endocrine regulation of the growth plate. Horm Res 64:157–165

106. Michael M, Jr C (2006) The New Bone Biology: Pathologic, Molecular, and Clinical Correlates. Am J Med Genet A 140A:2646–2706

107. Orth MW (1999) The regulation of growth plate cartilage turnover. J Anim Sci 77(Sup 2):183–189

108. Calmar EA, Vinci RJ (2002) The anatomy and physiology of bone fracture and healing. Clin Ped Emerg Med 3:85–93

109. Ballock TR, O'Keefe RJ (2003) Physiology and pathophysiology of the growth plate. Birth Defects Res 69:123–143

110. Dijkgraaf LC, De Bont LGM, Boering G, Liem RSB (1995) Normal cartilage structure, biochemistry, and metabolism: a review of the literature. J Oral Maxillofac Surg 53:924–929

111. Stevens DG, Boyer MI, Bowen CV (1999) Transplantation of epiphyseal plate allografts between animals of different ages. J Pediatr Orthop 19:398–403

112. Weise M, De-Levi S, Barnes KM, Gafni RI, Abad V, Baron J (2001) Effects of estrogen on growth plate senescence and epiphyseal fusion. Proc Natl Acad Sci USA 98:6871–6876

113. Gafni RI, Weise M, Robrecht DT, Meyers JL, Barnes KM, De Levi S, Baron J (2001) Catch-up growth is associated with delayed senescence of the growth plate in rabbits. Pediatr Res 50:618–623

114. Hoshi K, Ogata N, Shimoaka T, Terauchi Y, Kadowaki T, Kenmotsu S, Chung UI, Ozawa H, Nakamura K, Kawaguchi H (2004) Deficiency of insulin receptor substrate-1 impairs skeletal growth through early closure of epiphyseal cartilage. J Bone Miner Res 19:214–223

115. Philipps AF, Rosenkrantz TS, Clark RM, Knox I, Chaffin DG, Raye JR (1991) Effects of fetal insulin deficiency on growth in fetal lambs. Diabetes 40:20–27

116. Heinze E, Vetter U, Voigt KH (1989) Insulin stimulates skeletal growth in vivo and in vitro-comparison with growth hormone in rats. Diabbetologica 32:198–202

117. Vortkamp A, Lee K, Lanske B, Segre GV, Kronenberg HM, Tabin CJ (1996) Regulation of rate of cartilage differentiation by Indian hedgehog and PTH-related protein. Science 273: 613–622

118. Provot S, Schipani E (2005) Molecular mechanisms of endochondral bone development. Biophys Biochem Res Com 328:658–665

119. Kobayashi T, Soegiarto DW, Yang Y, Lanske B, Schipani E, McMahon AP, Kronenberg HM (2005) Indian hedgehog stimulates periarticular chondrocyte differentiation to regulate growth plate length independently of PTHrP. J Clin Invest 115:1734–1742

120. Kronenberg HM (2003) Developmental regulation of the growth plate. Nature 423: 332–336

121. Kronenberg HM (2006) PTHrP and skeletal development. Ann N Y Acad Sci 1068:1–13

122. Schwartz Z, Semba S, Graves D, Dean DD, Sylvia VL, Boyan BD (1997) Rapid and long-term effects of PTH (1–34) on growth plate chondrocytes are mediated through two different pathways in a cell-maturation-dependent manner. Bone 21:249–259

123. Spter D, Hill TP, O'Sullivan RJ, Gruber M, Conner DA, Hartmann C (2006) Wnt9a signaling is required for joint integrity and regulation of Ihh during chondrogenesis. Dev Dis 133: 3039–3049

124. Keenan BS, Richards GE, Ponder SW, Dallas JS, Nagamani M, Smith ER (1993) Androgen-stimulated pubertal growth: the effects of testosterone and dihydrotestosterone on growth hormone and insulin-like growth factor I in the treatment of short stature and delayed puberty. J Clin Endocrinol Metab 76:996–1001

125. Adams SL, Cohen AJ, Lassova L (2007) Integration of signaling pathways regulating chondrocyte differentiation during endochondral bone formation. J Cell Physiol 213:635–641

126. Guo J, Chung U, Yang D, Karsenty G, Bringhurst FR, Kronenberg HM (2006) PTH/PTHrP receptor delays chondrocyte hypertrophy via both Runx2-dependent and -independent pathways. Dev Biol 292:116–128

127. Schmid C, Steiner T, Froesch ER (1984) Insulin-like growth factor I supports differentiation of cultured osteoblast-like cells. FEBS Lett 173:48–52

128. Smink JJ, Koster JG, Gresnigt MG, Rooman R, Koedam JA, van Buul-Offers SC (2002) IGF and IGF-binding protein expression in the growth plate of normal, dexamethasone-treated and human IGF-II transgenic mice. J Endocrinol 175:143–153

129. Heinrichs C, Yanovski JA, Roth AH, Yu YM, Domene HM, Yano K, Cutler GB Jr, Baron J (1994) Dexamethasone increases growth hormone receptor messenger ribonucleic acid levels in liver and growth plate. Endocrinology 135:1113–1118

130. Jux C, Leiber K, Hugel U, Blum W, Ohlsson C, Klaus G, Mehls O (1998) Dexamethasone impairs growth hormone (GH)-stimulated growth by suppression of local insulin-like growth factor (IGF)-I production and expression of GH- and IGF-I-receptor in cultured rat chondrocytes. Endocrinology 139:3296–3305

131. Lazarus JE, Hegde A, Andrade AC, Nilsson O, Baron J (2007) Fibroblast growth factor expression in the postnatal growth plate. Bone 40:577–586

132. Ornitz DM, Xu J, Colvin JS, McEwen DG, MacArthur CA, Coulier F (1996) Receptor specificity of the fibroblast growth factor family. J Biol Chem 271:15292–15297

133. Smink JJ, Gresnigt MG, Hamers N, Koedam JA, Berger R, van Buul-Offers SC (2003) Short-term glucocorticoid treatment of prepubertal mice decreases growth and IGF-I expression in the growth plate. J Endocrinol 177:381–388

134. Tamamura Y, Otani T, Kanatani N, Koyama E, Kitagaki J, Komori T, Yamada Y, Costantini F, Wakisaka S, Pacifici M, Iwamoto M, Enomoto-Iwamoto M (2005) Developmental regulation

of Wnt/β-Catenin signals is required for growth plate assembly, cartilage integrity, and endochondral ossification. J Biol Chem 280:19185–19195

135. Perry MJ, McDougall KE, Hou SC (2008) Tobias JH Impaired growth plate function in bmp-6 null mice. Bone 42:216–225

136. Sasaki A, Taketomi T, Wakioka T, Kato R, Yoshimura A (2001) Identification of a dominant negative mutant of Sprouty that potentiates fibroblast growth factor- but not epidermal growth factor-induced ERK activation. J Biol Chem 276:36804–36808

137. Pogue R, Lyons K (2006) BMP signaling in the cartilage growth plate. Curr Top Dev Biol 76:1–48

138. Nilsson O, Chrysis D, Pajulo O, Boman A, Holst M, Rubinstein J, Martin RE, Savendahl L (2003) Localization of estrogen receptors-alpha and -beta and androgen receptor in the human growth plate at different pubertal stages. J Endocrinol 177:319–326

139. Lee K, Deeds JD, Bond AT, Juppner H, Abou-Samra AB, Segre GV (1993) In situ localization of PTH/PTHrP receptor mRNA in the bone of fetal and young rats. Bone 14:341–345

140. Lombard C, Nagarkatti M, Nagarkatti P (2007) CB2 cannabinoid receptor agonist, JWH-015, triggers apoptosis in immune cells: potential role for CB2-selective ligands as immunosuppressive agents. Clin Immunol 122:259–270

141. Wang Y, Nishida S, Sakata T, Elalieh HZ, Chang W, Halloran BP, Doty SB, Bikle DD (2006) Insulin-like growth factor-I is essential for embryonic bone development. Endocrinology 147:4753–4761

142. Gibson G (1998) Active role of chondrocyte apoptosis in endochondral ossification. Microsc Res Tech 43:191–204

143. Bar-Shavit Z (2007) The osteoclast: a multinucleated, hematopoietic-origin, bone resorbing osteoimmune cell. J Cell Biochem 102:1130–1139

144. Arron JR, Choi Y (2000) Bone versus immune system. Nature 408:535–536

145. Asagiri M, Takayanagi H (2007) The molecular understanding of osteoclast differentiation. Bone 40:251–264

146. Greenfield EM, Rubin J (2005) Osteoclast: origin and differentiation. In: Bronner F, Farach-Carson MC, Rubin J (eds) Bone resorption, vol 2, Topics in bone biology. Springer Science, Berlin, pp 1–23

147. Boyle WJ, Simonet WS, Lacey DL (2003) Osteoclast differentiation and activation. Nature 423:337–342

148. Miyamoto T, Ohneda O, Arai F, Iwamoto K, Okada S, Takagi K, Anderson DM, Suda T (2001) Bifurcation of osteoclasts and dendritic cells from common progenitors. Blood 98:2544–2554

149. Simonet WS, Lacey DL, Dunstan CR, Kelley M, Chang MS, Luthy R, Nguyen HQ, Wooden S, Bennett L, Boone T, Shimamoto G, DeRose M, Elliott R, Colombero A, Tan HL, Trail G, Sullivan J, Davy E, Bucay N, Renshaw-Gegg L, Hughes TM, Hill D, Pattison W, Campbell P, Sander S, Van G, Tarpley J, Derby P, Lee R, Boyle WJ (1997) Osteoprotegerin: a novel secreted protein involved in the regulation of bone density. Cell 89:309–319

150. Lacey DL, Timms E, Tan HL, Kelley MJ, Dunstan CR, Burgess T, Elliott R, Colombero A, Elliott G, Scully S, Hsu H, Sullivan J, Hawkins N, Davy E, Capparelli C, Eli A, Qian YX, Kaufman S, Sarosi I, Shalhoub V, Senaldi G, Guo J, Delaney J, Boyle WJ (1998) Osteoprotegerin ligand is a cytokine that regulates osteoclast differentiation and activation. Cell 93:165–176

151. Noble BS, Peet N, Stevens HY, Brabbs A, Mosley JR, Reilly GC, Reeve J, Skerry TM, Lanyon LE (2003) Mechanical loading: biphasic osteocyte survival and targeting of osteoclasts for bone destruction in rat cortical bone. Am J Physiol Cell Physiol 284:C934–C943

152. Heino TJ, Hentunen TA, Väänänen HK (2002) Osteocytes inhibit osteoblastic bone resorption through transforming growth factor b: enhancement by estrogen. J Cell Biochem 85:185–197

153. Delaisse JM, Andersen TL, Engsig MT, Henriksen K, Troen T, Blavier L (2003) Matrix metalloproteinases (MMP) and cathepsin K contribute differently to osteoclastic activities. Microsc Res Tech 61:504–513

154. Teitelbaum SL, Ross FP (2003) Genetic regulation of osteoclast development and function. Nat Rev Genet 4:638–649

155. Ross FP, Teitelbaum SL (2005) avb3 and macrophage colony-stimulating factor: partners in osteoclast biology. Immunol Rev 208:88–105
156. Gowen M, Lazner F, Dodds R, Kapadia R, Field J, Tavaria M, Bertoncello I, Drake F, Zavarselk S, Tellis I, Hertzog P, Debouck C, Kola I, Cathepsin K (1999) knockout mice develop osteopetrosis due to a deficit in matrix degradation but not demineralization. J Bone Miner Res 14:1654–1663
157. Mulari M, Vaaraniemi J, Vaananen HK (2003) Intracellular membrane trafficking in bone resorbing osteoclasts. Microsc Res Tech 61:496–503
158. McDonald MM, Dulai S, Godfrey C, Amanat N, Sztynda T, Little DG (2008) Bolus or weekly zoledronic acid administration does not delay endochondral fracture repair but weekly dosing enhances delays in hard callus remodeling. Bone 43:653–662

Chapter 3
Primary Mineralization

Jona J. Sela

3.1 Introduction

Primary mineralization in hard tissues is widely documented. Hydroxyapatite crystal (HA) formation in the matrix is regulated by forming cells (chondroblasts, osteoblasts, cementoblasts, and odonoblasts) and commonly initiated within extracellular matrix vesicles (MV). MVs, containing relatively high concentrations of Ca^{2+} and inorganic phosphate (Pi), are an optimal environment for hydroxyapatite crystallization. Alongside this process, a continuous mineralization of the matrix, without MVs, is evident. Concurrently, primary mineralization via MVs has been shown in the early stages of development in cartilage, bone, dentin, and cementum. Furthermore, it is well established that MVs serve as initial loci of calcification in tissues of mesenchymal origin not only in the embryonic stage but also during continuous growth as well as in bone repair and in mineralizing neoplastic conditions [1–25]. Primary mineralization was investigated by ultrastructural, biochemical, and molecular methods.

Proteomic analysis revealed that more than 60% of the total proteins were present in the cellular microvilli in human osteosarcoma cell line (Saos-2). Among all identified MV proteins, cytoskeletal markers of microvilli, including actin, ezrin, radixin, moesin, talin1, and actin-binding proteins such as cofilin1 and transgelin2, were present [26–28]. These findings support the observation that microvilli are the sites of origin of MVs and the finding that actin filament assembly and disassembly are involved in their biogenesis with a metabolically active outer membrane [16, 17, 19, 21, 22]. Vesicular release into the matrix is concomitant with their considerable loading with Ca^{2+} and Pi that produce calcifying foci on the vesicular inner membrane. Subsequent to exocytosis, MVs display high levels of enzymatic activity of alkaline phosphatase (AP), phospholipase-A$_2$ (PA$_2$),

J.J. Sela (✉)

Laboratory of Biomineralization, Institute of Dental Sciences, The Hebrew University
Hadassah – Faculty of Dental Medicine, P.O. Box 12272, Jerusalem 91120, Israel
e-mail: jjsela@cc.huji.ac.il

J.J. Sela and I.A. Bab (eds.), *Principles of Bone Regeneration*,
DOI 10.1007/978-1-4614-2059-0_3, © Springer Science+Business Media, LLC 2012

44 J.J. Sela

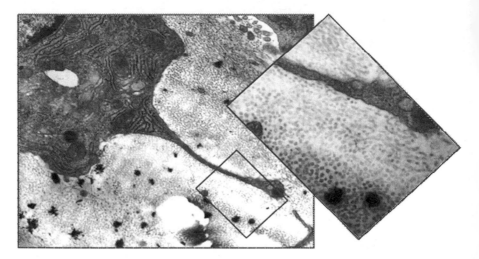

Fig. 3.1 Transmission electron micrograph of osteoblast with its process. *Insert*: Higher magnification. Note, vesicles in process and electron opaque vesicle in the matrix

pyrophosphatase (PP), different ATPases, and elevated contents of phosphatidylserine (PS). AP and annexins participate in the nucleation and formation of HA crystals. Annexins are Ca^{2+} and lipid-binding proteins involved in Ca^{2+} homeostasis in bone cells and MVs; they participate in the formation of calcium ion channel within the MV membrane. AP is associated with Pi regulation by hydrolysis of phosphate compounds. ATP and pyrophosphate, known inhibitors of HA formation, are hydrolyzed by AP, ATPases, and PP. In this respect, antagonistic activities serve in the regulation of the process of mineralization [16, 17, 19, 21, 22, 29, 30]. The process of bone healing is characterized by increased enzymatic activities and PS content on the first and second weeks after injury followed by a decreased activity on the third and fourth weeks. Quantitative-morphometric-ultrastructural studies demonstrated a typical gradient of vesicular distribution from the calcified front, with the ruptured MVs being the closest to the front, and the electron-lucent MVs being farthest away.

The biochemical and the ultrastructural observations clearly demonstrate the vesicular life cycle. Briefly, the vesicle is released from the osteoblast into the extracellular matrix in an electron-lucent form (Fig. 3.1). At this point AP is associated with Pi release in the matrix by hydrolysis of phosphate compounds. Annexins are responsible for influx of ionic calcium and phosphate that form saturated solutions of amorphous calcium-phosphate complexes producing MVs with an electron opaque texture (Fig. 3.2). ATP and pyrophosphate, the principal inhibitors of HA crystallization, are hydrolyzed by AP, ATPases, and PP, allowing intravesicular hydroxyapatite crystals formation (Fig. 3.3). Further crystal growth is accompanied by an increase in PA2 activity, resulting in rupture of the vesicular membranes and release of HA crystals to augment the calcifying fronts (Fig. 3.4) [31–39]. Schematic illustration of the process is summarized in Fig. 3.5.

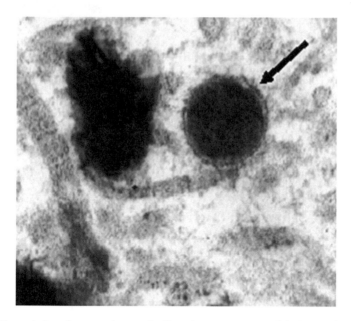

Fig. 3.2 Transmission electron micrograph of an electron opaque vesicle (*arrow*) in the matrix. Note, Collagen with cross banding (*left*) and a small calcospheritic structure constructed of HA crystals

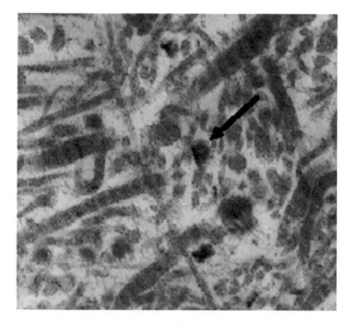

Fig. 3.3 Transmission electron micrograph of crystal containing vesicles (*arrow*) in collagen rich matrix

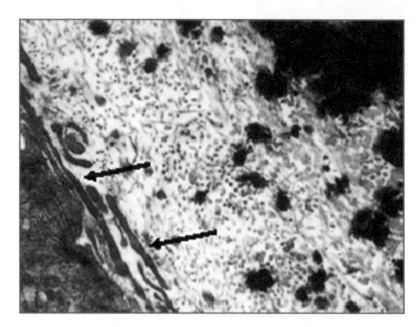

Fig. 3.4 Transmission electron micrograph of osteoblast with flattened processes (*arrows*) separated from the calcifying front (*black*) by collagenous matrix with dispersed calcospheritic structures

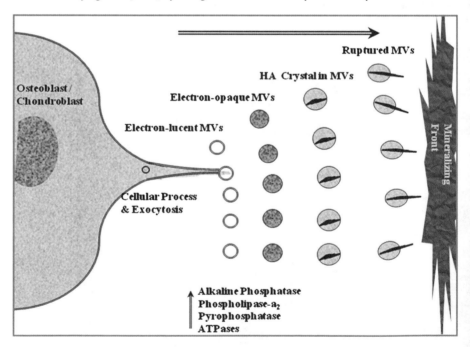

Fig. 3.5 Schematic illustration of MV mineralization process. The vesicle is released from the osteoblast or chondroblast into the extracellular matrix in an electron-lucent form. Increased AP is associated with Pi release in the matrix by hydrolysis of phosphate compounds. Annexins are responsible for influx of ionic calcium and phosphate that form saturated solutions of amorphous calcium-phosphate complexes producing MVs with an electron opaque texture. Intravesicular hydroxyapatite crystals formation and further crystal growth are accompanied by an increase in PA2 activity, resulting in rupture of the vesicular membranes and release of HA crystals that to augment the calcifying front

References

1. Bonucci E (1967) Fine structure of early cartilage calcification. J Ultrastruct Res 20:33–50
2. Anderson HC (1967) Electron microscopic studies of induced cartilage development and calcification. J Cell Biol 35:81–101
3. Anderson HC (1969) Vesicles associated with calcification in the matrix of epiphyseal cartilage. J Cell Biol 41:59–72
4. Bonucci E (1970) Fine structure and histochemistry of calcifying globules in epiphyseal cartilage from young rats. Z Zelleforsch Mikroks Anat 103:192–217
5. Ali SY, Evans L (1973) The uptake of Ca45 ions by matrix vesicles isolated from calcifying cartilage. Biochem J 134:647–651
6. Ali SY (1976) Analysis of matrix vesicles and their role in the calcification of epiphyseal cartilage. Fed Proc Am Soc Exp Biol 35:135–142
7. Ali SY, Wisby A, Gray JC (1977) The sequences of calcium and phosphorus accumulation by matrix vesicles. Calcif Tissue Res 22:490–493
8. Sela J, Bab I, Muhlrad A (1978) Ultrastructural and biochemical characterization of extracellular matrix vesicles in healing of alveolar bone sockets. Preliminary indications for the presence of contractile proteins. Metab Bone Dis Rel Res 1:185–191
9. Cecil RNA, Anderson HC (1978) Freeze structure studies of matrix vesicle calcification growth plate. Metab Bone Dis Rel Res 1:89–95
10. Hsu HHT, Anderson HC (1978) Calcification of isolated matrix vesicles from fetal cartilage. Proc Natl Acad Sci USA 75:3805–3808
11. Sela J, Bab I (1979) The relationship between extracellular matrix vesicles and calcospherites in primary mineralization of neoplastic bone tissue (TEM & SEM studies on osteosarcoma). Virchows Arch A Path Anat Histol 382:1–9
12. Sela J, Bab I (1979) Correlative transmission and scanning electron microscopy of the initial mineralization of healing alveolar bone in rats. Acta Anat 105:401–408
13. Ennever J, Vogel JJ (1980) Correlation of apatite nucleation and proteolipid integrity. J Dent Res 59:1175–1179
14. Ali SY (1980) Mechanism of calcification. In: Oven R, Goodfellow J, Bollough P (eds) Scientific foundations of orthopaedics and traumatology. Heinmann, London, pp 175–184
15. Sela J, Bab I, Muhlrad A (1981) A comparative study on the occurrence and activity of extracellular matrix vesicles in young and adult rat maxillary bone. Calcif Tissue Int 33:129–134
16. Muhlrad A, Bab I, Sela J (1981) Dynamic changes in bone cells and extracellular matrix vesicles during healing of alveolar bone in rats. Metab Bone Dis Rel Res 2:347–356
17. Sela J, Bab I, Muhlrad A, Stein M (1981) Extracellular matrix vesicles in human osteogenic neoplasms. Cancer 48:1602–1611
18. Ali SY, Evans L (1981) Mechanism of mineral formation by matrix vesicles. In: Ascenzi A, Bonucci E, Bernard B (eds) Proceedings of the 3rd international conference on matrix vesicles. Witchig, Milan, pp 67–72
19. Deutsch D, Bab I, Muhlrad A, Sela J (1982) Purification and further characterization of isolated matrix vesicles from rat alveolar bone. Metab Bone Dis Rel Res 3:209–214
20. Wuthier RE (1982) A review of primary mechanism of endochondral calcification with special emphasis on the role of cells mitochondria and matrix vesicles. Clin Orthop Rel Res 171:219–242
21. Muhlrad A, Setton A, Sela J, Bab I, Deutsch D (1983) Biochemical characterization of matrix vesicles from bone and cartilage. Metab Bone Dis Rel Res 5:93–99
22. Bab I, Deutsch D, Schwartz Z, Muhlrad A, Sela J (1983) Correlative morphometric and biochemical analysis of purified extracellular matrix vesicles from rat alveolar bone. Calcif Tissue Int 35:320–326
23. Lowe J, Bab I, Stein H, Sela J (1983) Primary calcification in remodeling Haversian system following tibial fracture in rats. Clin Orthop Relat Res 176:291–297
24. Ali SY (1983) Calcification of cartilage. In: Hall BK (ed) Cartilage, structure function and biochemistry, vol 1. Academic, Orlando, pp 343–378

25. Anderson HC, Mulhall D, Garimella R (2010) Role of extracellular membrane vesicles in the pathogenesis of various diseases, including cancer, renal diseases, atherosclerosis, and arthritis. Mini Rev Lab Invest 90:1549–1557
26. Thouverey C, Balcerzak M, Strzelecka-Kiliszek A, Pikula S, Buchet R (2008) Origin of matrix vesicles in mineralization competent osteoblast-like saos-2 cells. Bone 42(S1):S31–S32
27. Thouverey C, Strzelecka-Kiliszek A, Balcerzak M, Buchet R, Pikula S (2009) Matrix vesicles originate from apical membrane microvilli of mineralizing osteoblast-like Saos-2 cells. J Cell Biochem 106:127–138
28. Thouverey C, Balcerzak M, Strzelecka-Kiliszek A, Buchet R, Pikula S (2008) Apical microvilli of osteoblast-like SAOS-2 cells as precursors of calcifying matrix vesicles: a comparative proteomic study. CalcTissue Int 82 (Suppl):S120
29. Balcerzak M, Hamade E, Zhang L, Pikula S, Azzar G, Radisson J, Bandorowicz-Pikula J, Buchet R (2003) The roles of annexins and alkaline phosphatase in mineralization process. Acta Biochem Polon 50:1019–1038, Review
30. Thouverey C, Bechkoff G, Pikula S, Buchet R (2009) Inorganic pyrophosphate as a regulator of hydroxyapatite or calcium pyrophosphate dehydrate mineral deposition by matrix vesicles. Osteoarthritis Cartilage 17:1764–1772
31. Sela J, Amir D, Schwartz Z, Weinberg H (1987) Ultrastructural tissue morphometry of the distribution of extracellular matrix vesicles in remodeling rat tibial bone 6 days after injury. Acta Anat 128:295–300
32. Schwartz Z, Amir D, Weinberg H, Sela J (1987) Extracellular matrix vesicle distribution in primary mineralization 2 weeks after injury to rat tibial bone. Eur J Cell Biol 45:97–101
33. Sela J, Amir D, Schwartz Z, Weinberg H (1987) Changes in the distribution of extracellular matrix vesicles during healing of rat tibial bone (computerized morphometry and electron microscopy). Bone 8:245–250
34. Amir D, Schwartz Z, Sela J, Weinberg H (1988) The distribution of extracellular matrix vesicles in healing tibial bone 3 days after intramedullary injury. Arch Orthop Trauma Surg 107:1–6
35. Amir D, Schwartz Z, Sela J, Weinberg H (1988) The relationship between extracellular matrix vesicles and the calcifying front on the 21st day after injury to rat tibial bone. Clin Orthop 230:289–295
36. Schwartz Z, Sela J, Ramirez V, Amir D, Boyan BD (1989) Changes in extracellular matrix vesicles during healing of rat tibial bone: a morphometric and biochemical study. Bone 10:53–60
37. Sela J, Schwartz Z, Amir D, Swain LD, Boyan BD (1992) The effect of bone injury on extracellular matrix vesicle proliferation and mineral formation. Bone Miner 17:163–167
38. Sela J, Schwartz Z, Swain L, Amir D, Boyan BD (1992) Extracellular matrix vesicles in endochondral bone development and in healing after injury. Cells Mat 2:153–161
39. Sela J, Ornoy A (1995) Normal and abnormal primary mineralization. In: Ornoy A (ed) Animal models of human calcium metabolic disorders, vol 2. CRC, Boca Raton, pp 23–49

Part II
Systemic Factors in Bone Healing

Chapter 4
Anabolic Agents in Bone Repair

Itai A. Bab

Systemically administered bone anabolic agents that stimulate bone and cartilage formation in fracture healing have attracted much attention. These anabolic agents include parathyroid hormone (PTH), osteogenic growth peptide (OGP), statins, and vitamin D (Vit D).

PTH is an 84-amino acid polypeptide hormone secreted by the parathyroid glands. Its main function is to maintain extracellular calcium at normal levels by upregulating renal calcium and phosphate reabsorption, and bone resorption and release of calcium from the skeleton. It has been repeatedly demonstrated that all the known biological activities of PTH reside within the 1–34 N-terminal fragment. In experimental models of osteoporosis, intermittent treatment with PTH leads to the rescue of bone mass and mechanical strength consequent to increased osteoblastic activity. These anabolic effects are in contrast to the catabolic actions induced by continuous exposure to PTH. Teriparatide is a synthetic polypeptide hormone that consists of the 1–34 amino acid fragment of human PTH [rhPTH (1–34)]. It is used clinically to treat osteoporosis. Daily subcutaneous injections of teriparatide in osteoporotic patients stimulate cancellous bone formation, increase bone mineral density, and reduce the risk of fractures. Also, recombinant PTH (1–84) is used in the treatment of osteoporosis. Over the past several years, there has been an increasing interest in potential technologies for enhancing fracture healing. Part of this interest is derived from the growing age of the population and the recognition that increased age carries an increased risk of complications after fracture. Although use of locally implanted or injected growth factors has received the most attention, systemic treatments for the enhancement of bone repair, especially for situations in which bone repair may be diminished or delayed, are now under investigation. Since the approval of

I.A. Bab (✉)
Bone Laboratory, Institute of Dental Sciences, The Hebrew University of Jerusalem,
P.O. Box 12272, Jerusalem 91120, Israel
e-mail: babi@cc.huji.ac.il

J.J. Sela and I.A. Bab (eds.), *Principles of Bone Regeneration*,
DOI 10.1007/978-1-4614-2059-0_4, © Springer Science+Business Media, LLC 2012

teriparatide as an anabolic treatment for osteoporosis, there has been an increasing interest in other potential clinical uses for this compound, as well as other bone anabolic agents, in musculoskeletal conditions. Recently, a growing body of evidence has supported the conclusion that PTH (1–34) will also be an effective anabolic therapy for the enhancement of bone repair after fracture. Indeed, ongoing research has demonstrated the potential of PTH (1–34) in the management of bone repair in a number of bone healing models. In naive rodents, intermittent PTH (1–34) administration at doses of 30–200 μg/kg/day, initiated after fracture, stimulates the structural and biomechanical properties of the callus and enhances fracture healing. However, as PTH (1–34) is approved for anti-osteoporotic therapy, and because of the increased fracture risk in osteoporosis, it is also important to see if fractures occurring during ongoing PTH (1–34) treatment show a similar response. Indeed, PTH (1–34) pretreatment in rats does improve fracture healing unless supported by continuous treatment after fracture. Studies in cynomolgus monkeys, a species more closely related to humans, also showed acceleration of mid-femoral fracture healing by low-dose intermittent PTH (1–34) treatment. The above studies demonstrate the feasibility of using PTH, either the full length peptide or 1–34 amino terminal part, for the enhancement of regular fracture repair. Importantly, PTH has been shown to be effective also in experiment models for situations known to restrain bone healing such as aging, gonadal hormone deficiency, and malnutrition. Literature search could not reveal studies on the effect of PTH in animal models of critical size fracture nonunion. Clinical trial in humans showed that teriparatide shortened the time of healing of distal radial fractures in postmenopausal women by 2 weeks. Although this result means that PTH (1–34) may be effective in human, it has to be substantiated in trials involving more patients and additional skeletal sites [1–5].

OGP is a 14-amino acid chain identical to the C-terminal region of histone H4 (H4). It is produced by cells of the stromal lineage such as fibroblasts and osteoblasts and present in the blood circulation at micromolar concentrations. OGP and some of its naturally occurring and synthetic analogues have an established role as bone anabolic agents and hematopoietic stimulators. The discovery of OGP in the early 1990s followed the observation of enhanced systemic bone formation associated with post-ablation bone marrow regeneration [6]. A highly reproducible and controllable model system of experimental myelopoiesis occurs during regeneration of bone marrow after mechanical, chemical, or radioablation. Following such injuries, bone marrow regeneration is preceded by an intermediate phase of osteogenesis in which the affected medullary cavity is transiently filled with primary trabecular bone [7–10]. The intramedullary bone is resorbed and replaced by normal bone marrow. This osteogenic phase is accompanied by a systemic increase in bone formation [11]. OGP was initially isolated from primary bone during post-ablation healing bone marrow [12]. It regulates the local osteogenic response and transferred to the blood circulation and stimulates bone formation systemically [11–16]. OGP also promotes osteoblastic differentiation of bone marrow stromal stem cells through the stimulation of heme oxygenase-1 levels. It has been shown in vitro and in vivo that OGP levels are regulated by an autocrine/paracrine circuit as well as by binding

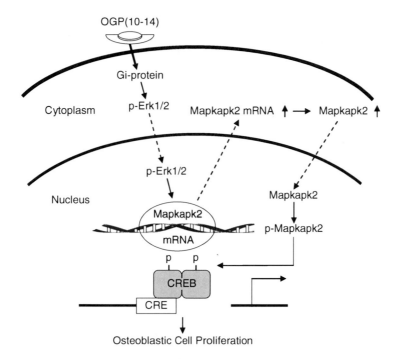

Fig. 4.1 OGP signaling. Following dissociation of the OGP–OGPBP complexes, the OGP is proteolytically processed in the extracellular milieu generating the active OGP. The formation of a putative OGP–OGP receptor complex leads to the activation of the intracellular Gi protein-CREB signaling cascade

to and dissociation from α2M. In rodents, exogenously administered OGP and OGP [12–17] stimulate osteoblastic activity and trabecular bone formation, thus preventing or reversing bone loss. The enhanced fracture healing was accompanied by elevated expression of genes involved in osteogenesis such as type II transforming growth factor-beta (TGF-β2), type I collagen, and the receptor for basic fibroblast growth factor [18, 19]. These studies suggest a role for OGP in the physiologic regulation of osteoblastic activity and bone mass and demonstrate its therapeutic potential as a bone anabolic agent for the systemic and local stimulation of bone formation. It has been demonstrated in osteoblasts that this pentapeptide binds to and activates a Gi protein-coupled receptor, which targets a mitogenic Erk1/2-Mapkapk2-CREB signaling pathway (Fig. 4.1) [20–26].

The biosynthesis of OGP is presented in Fig. 4.2. OGP is a H4 gene product. A pre-OGP is translated from H4 mRNA by a mechanism known as alternative translational initiation. The pre-OGP is proteolytically processed to become OGP. In the circulation, most of the OGP is present as a complex with α2-macroglobulin (α2M) thus being protected from proteolysis. Upon dissociation from α2M, the free OGP is proteolytically activated into its biologically active form, OGP [27–38].

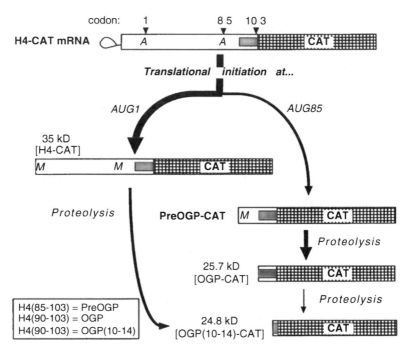

Fig. 4.2 Biosynthesis of OGP via alternative translational initiation at AUG85 of histone H4 mRNA. Pre-OGP [H4 (85–103)] is produced by alternative translational initiation at AUG85, and then proteolytically cleaved to yield OGP. OGP is slowly converted to OGP [i.e., H4 (99–103)], which, in addition, can be produced from full length H4 by proteolytic cleavage. The chloramphenicol acetyl transferase (CAT) derivatives are illustrated to directly reflect the actual data. A and M represent AUG codon and methionine residue, respectively. The correspondence of OGP-related sequences to H4 carboxyl terminal-derived peptides is presented in the *box* at the *lower left corner*

The increase in serum OGP after bone marrow ablation or acute blood loss is closely correlated with the enhancement of bone formation associated with these manipulations (Figs. 4.3 and 4.4). The OGP-induced increase in trabecular bone volume in these instances occurs consequent to an increase in trabecular thickness and connectivity. It has been demonstrated in rabbits and rats that systemically administered OGP stimulates fracture healing by enhancing the cartilage-to-bone transition in the fracture callus [39, 40].

Statins are 3-hydroxy-3-methylglutaryl (HMG)-CoA reductase inhibitors. They are anti-lipidemic, thus lowering cholesterol and reduce the incidence of cardiovascular disease. High doses of orally administered simvastatin have previously been shown to improve fracture healing in a mouse femur fracture model. In vitro and in vivo evidence could suggest that there are anabolic effects of statins in bone metabolism. Although evidence in patients with osteoporosis is conflicting, several studies have shown that the use of statins is associated with increases in bone mass density and reduction in fracture risk. The conflicting data may be due to different routes of administration, types of statins employed, and low doses used. In laboratory animals,

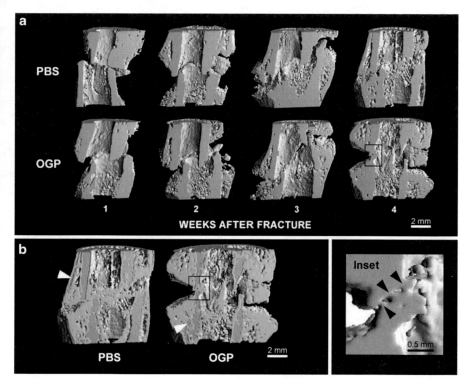

Fig. 4.3 Three-dimensional μCT images of fractured femora. (**a**) Effect of healing time and treatment on osseous components. *Inset*, high magnification of framed zone (4-week OGP). Note partially remodeled cortical union (*arrowheads*). (**b**) Overlay label of newly formed bone in specimens from 4-week OGP and control animals

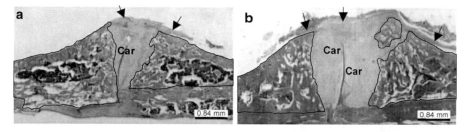

Fig. 4.4 Four-week fracture callus. (**a**) OGP-treated animal; (**b**) control animal. *Car*, cartilaginous callus; *contoured areas*, osseous callus; *arrows*, fibrous tissue. Hematoxylin and eosin

a positive effect on biomechanical parameters of fracture healing by simvastatin treatment was demonstrated following direct application at the fracture area. Statins have been shown to stimulate BMP2 transcription and bone formation. This raises the possibility that they could be useful for enhancing fracture repair. Observational studies in patients treated with oral statins for lipid lowering have been controversial.

The likely reason for their inconsistent effects is that the statin concentration reaching the periphery was too low after oral administration to produce a reproducible biologic effect. Taken together, there is sufficient evidence to suggest further clinical trials to establish the effect of statins on fracture healing [41–45].

Vitamin D. Adequate dietary intake of Vit D and calcium is essential to building and maintaining healthy bones. Animal studies have shown increased mechanical strength of the callous and other beneficial effects with Vit D treatment after a fracture. Given the few potentially harmful side effects, calcium and Vit D supplementation have long been advocated in an effort to augment bone healing. In the only trial reported in the literature on the role of Vit D and calcium supplementation was performed in treating osteoporotic women aged 78 years who had experienced an acute fracture of the proximal humerus. The primary outcome was the difference in bone mass density at the fracture site between the normal and osteoporotic. There was a significant difference in callous formation 6 weeks after fracture in the treatment group, but this was not sustained at 12 weeks. The clinical relevance of this study is questionable, even if applied to the study population, and it certainly cannot be generalized to other populations [46–48].

References

1. Andreassen TT, Ejersted C, Oxlund H (1999) Intermittent parathyroid hormone (1–34) treatment increases callus formation and mechanical strength of healing rat fractures. J Bone Miner Res 14:960–968
2. Andreassen TT, Fledelius C, Ejersted C, Oxlund H (2001) Increases in callus formation and mechanical strength of healing fractures in old rats treated with parathyroid hormone. Acta Orthop Scand 72:304–307
3. Komatsubara S, Mashiba T, Mori S (2009) Bone fracture and the healing mechanisms. The effect of human parathyroid hormone on fracture healing. Clin Calcium 19:660–666
4. Alexander JM, Bab I, Fish S, Mueller R, Uchiyama T, Gronowicz G, Nahounou M, Zhao Q, White DW, Chorev M, Gazit D, Rosenblatt M (2001) Human parathyroid hormone 1-34 reverses bone loss in ovariectomized mice. J Bone Miner Res 16:1665–1673
5. Barnes GL, Kakar S, Vora S, Morgan EF, Gerstenfeld LC, Einhorn TA (2008) Stimulation of fracture-healing with systemic intermittent parathyroid hormone treatment. J Bone Joint Surg Am 1:120–127
6. Bab I, Gazit D, Chorev M, Muhlrad A, Shteyer A, Greenberg Z, Namdar M, Khan AJ (1992) Histone H4-related osteogenic growth peptide (OGP): a novel circulating stimulator of osteoblastic activity. EMBO J 11:1867–1873
7. Amsel S, Maniatis A, Tavassoli M, Crosby WH (1969) The significance of intramedullary cancellous bone formation in the repair of bone marrow tissue. Anat Rec 164:101–111
8. Patt HM, Maloney MA (1975) Bone marrow regeneration after local injury: a review. Exp Hematol 3:135–148
9. Gerasimov YV, Chailakhyan RK (1978) Effect of marrow cavity curettage on bone marrow stromal cell precursors. Biull Eksp Biol Med 86:362–365
10. Bab I (1995) Post ablation bone marrow regeneration: an *in vivo* model to study differential regulation of bone formation and resorption. Bone 17:437S–441S
11. Bab I, Gazit D, Massarawa A, Sela J (1985) Removal of tibial marrow induces increased formation of bone and cartilage in rat mandibular condyle. Calcif Tissue Int 37:551–555

12. Einhorn TA, Simon G, Devlin VJ, Warman J, Sidhu SP, Vigorita VJ (1990) The osteogenic response to distant skeletal injury. J Bone Joint Surg Am 72:1374–1378

13. Mueller M, Schilling T, Minne HW, Ziegler R (1991) A systemic acceleratory phenomenon (SAP) accompanies the regional acceleratory phenomenon (RAP) during healing of a bone defect in the rat. J Bone Miner Res 6:401–410

14. Gazit D, Karmish M, Holzman L, Bab I (1990) Regenerating marrow induces systemic increase in osteo- and chondrogenesis. Endocrinology 126:2607–2613

15. Gazit D, Shteyer A, Bab I (1989) Further characterization of osteogenic-cell growth promoting activity derived from healing bone marrow. Connect Tissue Res 23:153–161

16. Bab I, Gazit D, Muhlrad A, Shteyer A (1988) Regenerating bone marrow produces a potent growth factor activity to osteogenic cells. Endocrinology 123:345–352

17. Sun YQ, Ashhurst DE (1998) Osteogenic growth peptide enhances the rate of fracture healing in rabbits. Cell Biol Int 22:313–319

18. Wozney JM, Rosen V, Byrne M, Celeste AJ, Moutsatsos I, Wang EA (1990) Growth factors influencing bone development. J Cell Sci Suppl 13:149–156

19. Touriol C, Roussigne M, Gensac MC, Prats H, Prats AC (2000) Alternative translation initiation of human fibroblast growth factor 2 mRNA controlled by its 3'-untranslated region involves a Poly(A) switch and a translational enhancer. J Biol Chem 275:19361–19367

20. Greenberg Z, Chorev M, Muhlrad A, Shteyer A, Namdar-Attar M, Casap N, Vidson M, Bab I (1995) Structural and functional characterization of osteogenic growth peptide from human serum: identity with rat and mouse horologes. J Clin Endocrinol Metab 80:2330–2335

21. Bab I, Smith E, Gavish H, Namdar-Attar M, Chorev M, Chen Y, Muhlrad A, Birnbaum MJ, Stein G, Frenkel B (1999) Biosynthesis of osteogenic growth peptide via alternative translational initiation at AUG85 of histone H4 mRNA. J Biol Chem 274:14474–14481

22. Bab I, Einhorn TA (1993) Regulatory role of osteogenic growth polypeptides in bone formation and hemopoiesis. Crit Rev Eukaryot Gene Expr 3:31–46

23. Bab I, Einhorn TA (1994) Polypeptide factors regulating osteogenesis and bone marrow repair. J Cell Biochem 55:358–365

24. Suva LJ, Seedor JG, Endo N, Quartuccio HA, Thompson DD, Bab I, Rodan GA (1993) Pattern of gene expression following rat tibial marrow ablation. J Bone Miner Res 8:379–388

25. Greenberg Z, Gavish H, Muhlrad A, Chorev M, Shteyer A, Attar-Namdar M, Tartakovsky A, Bab I (1997) Isolation of osteogenic growth peptide from osteoblastic MC3T3 E1 cell cultures and demonstration of osteogenic growth peptide binding proteins. J Cell Biochem 65:359–367

26. Miguel SM, Namdar-Attar M, Noh T, Frenkel B, Bab I (2005) ERK1/2-activated de novo Mapkapk2 synthesis is essential for osteogenic growth peptide mitogenic signaling in osteoblastic cells. J Biol Chem 11:37495–37502

27. Gavish H, Bab I, Tartakovsky A, Chorev M, Mansur N, Greenberg Z, Namdar-Attar M, Muhlrad A (1997) Human α_2-macroglobulin is an osteogenic growth peptide binding protein. Biochemistry 36:14883–14888

28. Doenecke D, Albig W, Bode C, Drabent B, Franke K, Gavenis K, Witt O (1997) Histones: genetic diversity and tissue-specific gene expression. Histochem Cell Biol 107:1–10

29. Bab I, Muhlrad A, Chorev M, Shteyer A, Greenberg Z, Mansur N (1998) Osteogenic growth oligopeptides and pharmaceutical compositions containing them. US Patent 5, 814,610

30. Bab I, Gavish H, Namdar-Attar M, Muhlrad A, Greenberg Z, Chen Y, Mansur N, Shteyer A, Chorev M (1999) Isolation of mitogenically active c-terminal truncated pentapeptide of osteogenic growth peptide from human plasma and culture medium of murine osteoblastic cells. J Pept Res 54:408–414

31. Gabarin N, Gavish H, Muhlrad A, Chen YC, Namdar-Attar M, Nissenson RA, Chorev M, Bab I (2001) Mitogenic G_i protein-MAP kinase signaling cascade in MC3T3 E1 osteogenic cells: activation by C-terminal pentapeptide of osteogenic growth peptide [OGP(10-14)] and attenuation of activation by cAMP. J Cell Biochem 81:594–603

32. Greenberg Z, Chorev M, Muhlrad A, Shteyer A, Namdar M, Mansur N, Bab I (1993) Mitogenic action of osteogenic growth peptide (OGP): role of amino and carboxy terminal regions and charge. Biochim Biophys Acta 1178:273–280

33. Chen YC, Bab I, Mansur N, Muhlrad A, Shteyer A, Namdar-Attar M, Gavish H, Vidson M, Chorev M (2000) Structure-bioactivity of C-terminal truncated pentapeptide of osteogenic growth peptide [OGP(10-14)]. J Pept Res 56:147–156

34. Chen YC, Muhlrad A, Shteyer A, Vidson M, Bab I, Chorev M (2002) Bioactive pseudopeptidic analogues and cyclostereoisomers of osteogenic growth peptide C-terminal pentapeptide, OGP (10-14). J Med Chem 45:1624–1632

35. Goodman M, Chorev M (1979) On the concept of linear modified retro-peptide structures. Acc Chem Res 12:1–7

36. Chorev M, Goodman M (1993) A dozen years of retro-inverso peptidomimetics. Acc Chem Res 26:266–273

37. Fazzi R, Testi R, Trasciatti S, Galimberti S, Rosini S, Piras F, L'Abbate G, Conte A, Petrini M (2002) Bone and bone-marrow interactions: hematological activity of osteoblastic growth peptide (OGP)-derived carboxy-terminal pentapeptide. Mobilizing properties on white blood cells and peripheral blood stem cells in mice. Leuk Res 26:19–27

38. Fazzi R, Pacini S, Testi R, Azzarà A, Galimberti S, Testi C, Trombi L, Metelli MR, Petrini M (2003) Carboxy-terminal fragment of osteogenic growth peptide in vitro increases bone marrow cell density in idiopathic myelofibrosis. Br J Haematol 121:76–85

39. Robinson D, Bab I, Nevo Z (1995) Osteogenic growth peptide (OGP) regulates proliferation and osteogenic maturation of human and rabbit bone marrow stromal cells. J Bone Miner Res 10:690–696

40. Gabet Y, Muller R, Regev E, Sela J, Shteyer A, Salisbury K, Chorev M, Bab I (2004) Osteogenic growth peptide modulates fracture callus structural and mechanical properties. Bone 35:65–73

41. Skoglund B, Aspenberg P (2007) Locally applied Simvastatin improves fracture healing in mice. BMC Musculoskelet Disord 27:98

42. Gutierrez GE, Edwards JR, Garrett IR, Nyman JS, Mccluskey B, Rossini G, Flores A, Neidre DB, Mundy GR (2008) Transdermal lovastatin enhances fracture repair in rats. J Bone Miner Res 23:1722–1730

43. Chissas D, Stamatopoulos G, Verettas D, Kazakos K, Papalois A, Agrogiannis G, Papaeliou A, Agapitos E, Balanika A, Papadopoulou E, Anastopoulos G, Ntagiopoulos PG, Asimakopoulos A (2010) Can low doses of simvastatin enhance fracture healing? An experimental study in rabbits. Injury 41:687–692

44. Tang QO, Tran GT, Gamie Z, Graham S, Tsialogiannis E, Tsiridis E, Linder T, Tsiridis E (2008) Statins: under investigation for increasing bone mineral density and augmenting fracture healing. Expert Opin Investig Drugs 17:1435–1463

45. Patil S, Holt G, Raby N, Mclellan AR, Smith K, O'Kane S, Beastall G, Crossan JF (2009) Prospective, double blind, randomized, controlled trial of simvastatin in human fracture healing. J Orthop Res 27:281–285

46. Delgado-Martinez AD, Martinez ME, Carrascal MT, Rodriguez-Avial M, Munuera L (1998) Effect of 25-OH-vitamin D on fracture healing in elderly rats. J Orthop Res 16:650–653

47. Cao Y, Mori S, Mashiba T, Kaji Y, Manabe T, Iwata K, Miyamoto K, Komatsubara S, Yamamoto T (2007) 1Alpha, 25-dihydroxy-2beta(3-hydroxypropoxy)vitamin D3 (ED-71) suppressed callus remodeling but did not interfere with fracture healing in rat femora. Bone 40:132–139

48. Koester MC, Spindler KP (2006) Pharmacologic agents in fracture healing. Clin Sport Med 5:63–73

Chapter 5
Bone Repair in Diabetes

Gail Amir

Abstract Diabetes is associated with an increased risk of fracture of bone and impaired fracture healing. Wound complications are more serious and the rate of postoperative complications is higher than that in non diabetic subjects. The etiology and pathogenesis of impaired bone repair in human subjects and animal models of type I and type II diabetes are reviewed. In addition the adequacy of bone repair around orthopedic and dental implants is addressed and a role for hyperglycosylation in impaired bone repair in diabetic subjects is discussed.

5.1 Delayed Fracture Healing in Diabetes Mellitus

In general, osseous fracture is repaired to an extent that morphologically and functionally the original bone is restored. A sequential cascade of events occurs which can be divided into four overlapping histological stages. The inflammatory stage begins with hematoma formation at the site of the fracture. The hematoma is invaded by neutrophils and macrophages that digest and remove debris and then by fibroblasts that form a collagenous framework. In the second stage (soft callus formation) progenitors are recruited to the fracture site where they proliferate and differentiate into chondrocytes and osteoblasts. Chondrocytes produce cartilage giving rise to the soft fibrocartilagenous callus. The cartilage mineralizes and then undergoes apoptosis and is removed by osteoclasts. Hard callus formation occurs by osteoblastic proliferation giving rise to bony replacement of the fibrocartilagenous callus. The bony callus then undergoes remodeling by cycles of resorption and bone formation until the original architecture of the bone is restored [1]. At the cellular level, inflammatory cells, vascular cells, osteochondral progenitors, and osteoclasts

G. Amir (✉)
Hadassah Faculty of Medicine, Department of Pathology,
Hebrew University, Jerusalem, Israel
e-mail: gails@cc.huji.ac.il

J.J. Sela and I.A. Bab (eds.), *Principles of Bone Regeneration*,
DOI 10.1007/978-1-4614-2059-0_5, © Springer Science+Business Media, LLC 2012

are the key players in the repair process. At the molecular level, fracture repair is driven by three main classes of factors: pro-inflammatory cytokines and growth factors, pro-osteogenic factors, and angiogenic factors [2].

Diabetes has been shown to cause osteopenia, particularly in patients with type 1 diabetes, and is associated with an increased risk of fracture of the hip, proximal humerus and foot, and significantly impaired fracture healing in humans and in animal models of type 1 and type 2 diabetes [3–7]. The literature on the effects of DM on fracture healing in man pertains almost exclusively to healing of lower limb and ankle fractures. Delayed union is seen in displaced fractures of the lower extremity in type 1 and type 2 diabetic patients [6], and diabetes is a risk factor for nonunion of ankle fractures [8]. Fractures in diabetic patients treated surgically have a higher incidence of prolonged union time and serious wound complications compared to nondiabetic patients [9], and the overall rate of postoperative complications of fracture is higher [10]. Insights into the mechanisms of diabetes-induced delayed fracture healing come mainly from the study of animal models. Delayed and impaired healing of fractures has been observed in several models of type I diabetes. In 1965, Wray first demonstrated that the tensile strength of fracture callus in diabetic rats is significantly reduced compared to that in nondiabetic rats [7]. More recent studies confirm delayed recovery of structural strength [11] and decreased mechanical strength of fractures in diabetic rodent models [12]. Histological studies of animal models of DM have demonstrated evidence of delayed fracture callus formation characterized by reduced early cellular proliferation, delayed chondrogenesis [12–14], and reduced vascular response, corresponding with impaired mechanical tensile strength of the bone [12, 14–16]. The etiology and pathogenesis of poor fracture healing in diabetic patients are largely unknown and are probably multifactorial. Diabetic patients have an increased susceptibility to infection, and they frequently have comorbidities that impair fracture healing such as macro- and microangiopathy and neuropathy [8]. Diabetic neuropathy may contribute to impaired blood flow as well as to inappropriate weight bearing before adequate union is achieved [9]. In view of the complex cascade of events contributing to fracture repair and the multifaceted interactions of DM and bone metabolism, it is difficult to assess the significance of the contribution of any single dysfunction to the impairment of fracture healing.

A wealth of literature has accumulated implicating various etiologic factors in the disturbances of callus formation in diabetic subjects. These include hypoinsulinemia, hyperglycemia, increased oxidative stress, increased cell death, and inappropriate levels of growth factors at the site of the fracture.

Insulin has an anabolic effect on bone [17]. Hypoinsulinemia has been implicated in delayed fracture healing. Systemic insulin treatment reverses impaired bone healing in diabetic animals [18, 19]. Local delivery of insulin to a fracture site ameliorates fracture repair in diabetic rats without affecting blood glucose levels, indicating a direct effect of insulin on fracture healing [20]. Some studies suggest that many of the defects of fracture healing in diabetic models are a direct result of hyperglycemia. Impaired collagen synthesis by osteoblasts and chondroblasts correlates with the degree of hyperglycemia in diabetic models and is thought to play a major role in the impairment of callus formation. Blood glucose control in this model results in improved cellular proliferation and fracture healing and in normalized tensile strength [14, 15]. On the molecular level, high glucose levels modulate osteoblast gene expression resulting in bone loss and impaired osteoclast differentiation and function in vitro [21, 22]. This may be due to increased formation of advanced glycation endproducts (AGEs) induced by systemic hyperglycemia, possibly mediated through the AGE cell surface receptor, RAGE, on osteoblasts [23]. Oxidative stress is due to overproduction of reactive oxygen species (ROS). Increased oxidative stress is induced by a variety of mechanisms in diabetes, and it has been proposed as one of the major mechanisms of the hyperglycemia-induced trigger of diabetic complications [24]. Oxidative stress has been shown to inhibit osteoblast differentiation, to induce apoptosis of osteoblasts [25–27], to accelerate destruction of calcified tissue by osteoclasts, and is associated with a low turnover osteopenia. These changes can be reversed by administering antioxidants [28, 29]. The WNT pathway is involved in glucose homeostasis, and one of its functions is the regulation of differentiation of mesenchymal stem cells to osteoblasts or adipose cells, mediated by ß-catenin. It has been proposed that oxidative stress antagonizes the anabolic skeletal effects of Wnt/ß-catenin by diverting the limited pool of ß-catenin to FOXO-mediated transcription in osteoblasts [30, 31]. The FOXOs serve as a defense mechanism against oxidative damage by inducing cell cycle arrest and quiescence. Treatment with an antioxidant or with insulin suppresses oxidative stress and is associated with reversal of diabetes-associated osteopenia [32]. These findings suggest a role for oxidative stress in diabetic bone disease and may lead to the development of pharmacotherapeutic strategies to deal with impaired bone formation in diabetes [32, 33].

Impaired cartilage formation during fracture healing has been described in diabetic animals. They develop smaller fracture calluses than do nondiabetic animals during the period of transition from cartilage to bone, associated with increased cartilage resorption due to apoptosis of chondrocytes and increased osteoclastogenesis [34]. This contributes to impaired fracture healing by decreasing the scaffold for endochondral new bone formation [35]. The increased apoptotic rate of chondrocytes and increased osteoclastogenesis are normalized by insulin therapy, indicating that the adverse effects on fracture healing are directly related to the diabetic condition. Release of growth factors and cytokines at the fracture site is critical for organization and maturation of the early callus. Studies on diabetic rats have demonstrated decreased levels of platelet-derived growth factor (PDGF), transforming growth factor β (TGF-β), insulin-like growth factor I (IGF-I), vascular endothelial growth factor (VEGF), in early fracture callus associated with decreased cellular proliferation and impairment of collagen and extracellular matrix production, chondrocyte proliferation/differentiation and new blood vessel formation [13, 15, 36]. Local application of recombinant PDGF reverses these effects leading to enhanced fracture healing [37]. Low levels of expression of collagen type II, type X, and osteopontin have also been observed in diabetic rat callus [38]. Other studies implicate both the inflammatory stage and the soft callus stage. Inadequate callus formation and enhanced removal of cartilage from the callus in diabetic rats may be explained on a molecular level by the elevated levels of mRNA expression for aggrecanases that degrade cartilage (ADAMTS-4 and ADAMTS-5) and for cytokines that induce osteoclastogenesis

(TNF-α, M-CSF, RANKL, VEGF-A) [34, 35]. The impaired callus formation and the increased levels of cytokines are both reversed by insulin therapy. The final bone forming and remodeling stage of callus formation may also be impaired in diabetic subjects. Marrow ablation in diabetic mice is followed by reduced bone formation associated with reduced expression of critical transcription factors Runx2 and Dlx5 that regulate osteoblastic differentiation [39]. RANKL, its receptor RANK, and osteoprotegerin (OPG) provide the cellular and molecular basis for osteoblast–osteoclast cross talk which is crucial during bone remodeling. Interaction between RANK and RANKL on osteoclast precursors induces osteoclast differentiation leading to bone resorption. OPG is a decoy receptor of RANKL that antagonizes osteoclast differentiation. An imbalance between RANKL and OPG occurs at the fracture site in diabetic rats and may contribute to the delayed fracture repair in the diabetic condition [40].

Patients with diabetes have a higher complication rate after fracture. In addition to malunion, delayed union, and nonunion, these patients are also at risk for impaired wound healing, infection, and Charcot arthropathy. The latter is commoner in patients who were initially undiagnosed and had a delay in immobilization and in patients treated nonsurgically for displaced fractures [41]. There are many options for nonoperative and operative treatment of fractures in diabetic subjects. Correct soft tissue management and stable, rigid fixation with prolonged immobilization and prolonged restricted weight bearing are required in order to minimize problems and restore full function, particularly in patients with vasculopathy or neuropathy [42]. Regardless of whether insulin has a direct effect on fracture healing or whether its primary effect is to reverse hyperglycemia, the importance of managing serum glucose levels during fracture healing has been stressed by many investigators [14, 15, 34]. A better understanding of the cellular and molecular mechanisms of delayed fracture healing is expected to provide the basis for a new generation of drugs in the future to help promote fracture healing in diabetic subjects.

5.2 Delayed Bone Healing Around Orthopedic and Dental Implants in Diabetic Subjects

Diabetic patients undergoing arthroplasty have a higher rate of postoperative complications, particularly wound, medical, and orthopedic complications. They also have a higher revision rate and lower postoperative function scores than nondiabetic patients [43]. In addition, the long-term clinical results are worse than those of a control population due to the associated systemic complications of diabetic patients. Nevertheless, the long-term probability of implant survival is no different from that of nondiabetic subjects [44–46].

Assessment of the degree of osteointegration around metallic dental implants in experimental models of diabetes has given rise to conflicting reports. In many experimental models of type I diabetes, there is a reduced bone formation and reduced level of bone-implant contact. These changes are reversed after institution of insulin therapy, and they do not develop in insulin-controlled diabetic rats [47–50]. In other studies of insulin-dependant rats impaired osteointegration has been noted, but this was associated with increased bone response around the implant [51, 52]. The results of studies on osteointegration of implants in type II diabetes models are also contradictory. There are some reports of impaired bone-implant contact [53] while others have not found significant differences in osteointegration or trabecular bone volume around implants [54]. Diabetes is not a contraindication to dental implant placement [55]. Nevertheless, a higher failure rate of dental implants is seen in type I diabetic subjects compared to nondiabetic subjects. Most of these occur in the first year of functional loading, suggesting microvascular complications as a possible etiologic factor [48]. Increased liability to infection is another factor. Diabetic subjects have a higher incidence of bacterial-induced mucositis (soft tissue inflammation) and peri-implantitis (associated with bone loss) [56]. Good control of serum glucose levels has been shown to improve implant survival. Type II diabetes does not impact on dental implant survival or complication rate [57].

5.3 The Role of Hyperglycosylation

It has been proposed that chemical modification of proteins in diabetes alters the structure and function of tissue proteins giving rise to AGEs. AGEs are slowly and irreversibly formed on proteins exposed to carbonyl and substrate stress, especially in conditions of prolonged hyperglycemia, hyperlipidemia, and/or oxidative stress. The main targets for AGE formation are long-lived proteins such as collagen. Accumulation of AGE has been implicated in the development of long-term complications in diabetic subjects such as reduced elasticity and increased permeability of blood vessels [58]. AGE-mediated collagen cross linking can cause loss of flexibility and elasticity and increased brittleness of tissues like bone [59]. Long-term exposure to AGE-modified proteins has been shown to inhibit proliferation, differentiation, and mineralization of osteoblastic cultures while increasing apoptosis of osteoblasts and ROS production [60–62]. In addition, osteoclastogenesis is enhanced by upregulation of RANKL [63]. These changes are mediated via specific receptors for AGE on osteoblasts (RAGE) [23, 64, 65]. This mechanism is thought to play an important role in the reduced strength, increased fracture risk, and impaired bone healing in diabetes and may in the future prove to be a useful drug target [60, 66].

References

1. Kagel EM, Einhorn TA (1996) Alterations of fracture healing in the diabetic condition. Iowa Orthop J 16:147–152
2. Schindeler A, McDonald MM, Bokko P, Little DG (2008) Bone remodeling during fracture repair. The cellular picture. Semin Cell Dev Biol 19:459–466
3. Schwartz AV (2003) Diabetes mellitus: does it affect bone? Calcif Tissue Int 73:515–519

4. Tuominen JT, Impivaara O, Puukka P, Rönnemaa T (1999) Bone mineral density in patients with type 1 and type 2 diabetes. Diabetes Care 22:1196–1200
5. Macey LR, Kana SM, Jingushi S, Terek RM, Borretos J, Bolander ME (1989) Defects of early fracture-healing in experimental diabetes. J Bone Joint Surg Am 71:722–733
6. Loder R (1988) The influence of diabetes mellitus on the healing of closed fractures. Clin Orthop Relat Res 232:210–216
7. Wray JB, Stunkle E (1965) The effect of experimental diabetes upon the breaking strength of the healing fracture in the rat. J Surg Res 11:479–481
8. Wukich DK, Kline AJ (2008) The management of ankle fractures in patients with diabetes. J Bone Joint Surg Am 90:1570–1578
9. McCormack RG, Leith JM (1998) Ankle fractures in diabetics. Complications of surgical management. J Bone Joint Surg Br 80:689–692
10. Blotter RH, Connolly E, Wasan A, Chapman MW (1999) Acute complications in the operative treatment of isolated ankle fractures in patients with diabetes mellitus. Foot Ankle Int 20:687–694
11. Funk JR, Hale JE, Carmines D, Gooch HL, Hurwitz SR (2000) Biomechanical evaluation of early fracture healing in normal and diabetic rats. J Orthop Res 18:126–132
12. Gooch HL, Hale JE, Fujioka H, Balian G, Hurwitz SA (2000) Alterations of cartilage and collagen expression during fracture healing in experimental diabetes. Connect Tissue Res 41:81–91
13. Tyndall WA, Beam HA, Zarro C, O'Connor JP, Lin SS (2003) Decreased platelet derived growth factor expression during fracture healing in diabetic animals. Clin Orthop Relat Res 408:319–330
14. Herbsman H, Powers JC, Hirschman A, Shaftan GW (1968) Retardation of fracture healing in experimental diabetes. J Surg Res 8:424–431
15. Beam HA, Parsons JR, Lin SS (2002) The effects of blood glucose control upon fracture healing in the BB Wistar rat with diabetes mellitus. J Orthop Res 20:1210–1216
16. Harris BH, Powers J, Shaftan GW, Herbsman H (1968) Vascular component of fracture healing in experimental diabetes. Surg Forum 19:450–451
17. Thrailkill KM, Lumpkin CK Jr, Bunn RC, Kemp SF, Fowlkes JL (2005) Is insulin an anabolic agent in bone? Dissecting the diabetic bone for clues. Am J Physiol Endocrinol Metab 289:E735–E745
18. Klöting L, Follak N, Klöting I (2005) Diabetes per se and metabolic state influence gene expression in tissue-dependent manner of BB/OK rats. Diabetes Metab Res Rev 21:281–287
19. Follak N, Klöting L, Wolf E, Merk H (2004) Delayed remodeling in the early period of fracture healing in spontaneously diabetic BB/OK rats depending on the diabetic metabolic state. Histol Histopathol 19:473–486
20. Gandhi A, Beam HA, O'Conner JP, Parsons JR, Lin SS (2005) The effect of local insulin delivery on diabetic fracture healing. Bone 37:482–490
21. Wittrant Y, Gorin Y, Woodruff K, Horn D, Abboud HE, Mohan S, Abboud-Werner S (2008) High d(+)glucose concentration inhibits RANKL-induced osteoclastogenesis. Bone 42:1122–1130
22. Botolin S, McCabe LR (2006) Chronic hyperglycemia modulates osteoblast gene expression through osmotic and non-osmotic pathways. J Cell Biochem 99:411–424
23. Ogawa N, Yamaguchi T, Yano S, Yamauchi M, Yamamoto M, Sugimoto T (2007) The combination of high glucose and advanced glycation end-products (AGEs) inhibits the mineralization of osteoblastic MC3T3-E1 cells through glucose-induced increase in the receptor for AGEs. Horm Metab Res 39:871–875
24. Valko M, Leibfritz D, Moncol J, Cronin MT, Mazur M, Telser J (2007) Free radicals and antioxidants in normal physiological functions and human disease. Int J Biochem Cell Biol 39:44–84
25. Park YG, Kim KW, Song KH, Lee JM, Hong JJ, Moon SK, Kim CH (2009) Combinatory responses of proinflammatory cytokines on nitric-oxide mediated function in mouse calvarial osteoblasts. Cell Biol Int 33:92–99

26. Chen RM, Wu GJ, Chang HC, Chen JT, Chen TF, Lin YL, Chen TL (2005) 2,6-Diisopropylphenol protects osteoblasts from oxidative stress-induced apoptosis through suppression of caspase-3 activation. Ann NY Acad Sci 1042:448–459

27. Bai XC, Lu D, Bai J, Zheng H, Ke ZY, Li XM, Luo SQ (2004) Oxidative stress inhibits osteo-blastic differentiation of bone cells by ERK and NF-kappaB. Biochem Biophys Res Commun 314:197–207

28. Jagger CJ, Lean JM, Davies JT, Chambers TJ (2005) Tumor necrosis factor-alpha mediates osteopenia caused by depletion of antioxidants. Endocrinology 146:113–118

29. Lean JM, Davies JT, Fuller K, Jagger CJ, Kirstein B, Partington GA, Urry ZL, Chambers TJ (2003) A crucial role for thiol antioxidants in estrogen-deficiency bone loss. J Clin Invest 112:915–923

30. Jin T, The WNT (2008) Signalling pathway and diabetes mellitus. Diabetologia 51:1771–1780

31. Manolagas SC, Almeida M (2007) Gone with the Wints: beta-catenin, T-cell factor, forkhead box O, and oxidative stress in age-dependent diseases of bone, lipid and glucose metabolism. Mol Endocrinol 21:2605–2614

32. Hamada Y, Fujii H, Kitazawa R, Yodoi J, Kitazawa S, Fukagawa M (2009) Thioredoxin-1 overexpression in transgenic mice attenuates streptozotocin-induced diabetic osteopenia: a novel role of oxidative stress and therapeutic implications. Bone 44:936–941

33. Sheweita SA, Khoshhal KI (2007) Calcium metabolism and oxidative stress in bone fractures: role of antioxidants. Curr Drug Metab 8:519–525

34. Kayal RA, Alblowi J, McKenzie E, Krothapalli N, Silkman L, Gerstenfeld L, Einhorn TA, Graves DT (2009) Diabetes caused the accelerated loss of cartilage during fracture repair wgich is reversed by insulin treatment. Bone 44:357–363

35. Kayal RA, Tsatsas D, Bauer MA, Allen B, Al-Sebaei MO, Kakar S, Leone CW, Morgan EF, Gerstenfeld LC, Einhorn TA, Graves DT (2007) Diminished bone formation during diabetic fracture healing is related to the premature resorption of cartilage associated with increased osteoclast activity. J Bone Miner Res 22:560–568

36. Gandhi A, Doumas C, O'Connor JP, Parsons JR, Lin SS (2006) The effects of local plasma rich delivery on diabetic fracture healing. Bone 38:540–546

37. Al-Zube L, Breitbart EA, O'Connor JP, Parsons JR, Bradica G, Hart CE, Lin SS (2009) Recombinant human platelet-derived growth factor BB (rhPDGF-BB) and beta-tricalcium phosphate/collagen matrix enhance fracture healing in a diabetic rat model. J Orthop Res 27:1074–1081

38. Ogasawara A, Nakajima A, Nakajima F, Goto K, Yamazaki M (2008) Molecular basis for affected cartilage formation and bone union in fracture healing of the streptozotocin-induced diabetic rat. Bone 43:832–839

39. Lu H, Kraut D, Gerstenfeld LC, Graves DT (2003) Diabetes interferes with the bone formation by affecting the expression of transcription factors that regulate osteoblast differentiation. Endocrinology 144:345–352

40. de Amorim FP, Ornelas SS, Diniz SF, Batista AC, da Silva TA (2008) Imbalance of RANK, RANKL and OPG expression during tibial fracture repair in diabetic rats. J Mol Histol 39:401–408

41. Chaudhary SB, Liporace FA, Gandhi A, Donley BG, Pinzur MS, Lin SS (2008) Complications of ankle fracture in patients with diabetes. J Am Acad Orthop Surg 16:159–170

42. Gandhi A, Liporace F, Azad V, Mattie J, Lin SS (2006) Diabetic fracture healing. Foot Ankle Clin 11:805–824

43. Meding JB, Reddleman K, Keating ME, Klay A, Ritter MA, Faris PM, Berend ME (2003) Total knee replacement in patients with diabetes mellitus. Clin Orthop Relat Res 416:208–216

44. Bolognesi MP, Marchant MH Jr, Viens MA, Cook C, Pietrobon R, Vail TP (2008) The impact of diabetes on perioperative patient outcomes after total hip and total knee arthroplasty in the United States. J Arthroplasty 23(6 Suppl):92–98

45. Moon HK, Han CD, Yang IH, Cha BS (2008) Factors affecting outcome after total knee arthro-plasty in patients with diabetes mellitus. Yonsei Med J 49:129–137

46. Papagelopoulos PJ, Idusuyi OB, Wallrichs SL, Morrey BF (1996) Long term outcome and survivorship analysis of primary total knee arthroplasty in patients with diabetes mellitus. Clin Orthop Relat Res 330:124–132
47. de Morais JA, Trindade-Suedam IK, Pepato MT, Marcantonio E Jr, Wenzel A, Scaf G (2009) Effect of diabetes mellitus and insulin therapy on bone density around osseointegrated dental implants: a digital subtraction radiography study in rats. Clin Oral Implants Res 20:796–801
48. Mellado-Valero A, Ferrer Garcia C, Herrera Ballester A, Labuaig Rueda C (2007) Effects of diabetes on the osteointegration of dental implants. Med Oral Patol Oral Cir Bucal 12:E38–E43
49. Kwon PT, Rahan SS, Kim DM, Kopman JA, Karimbux NY, Fiorellini JP (2005) Maintenance of osseointegration utilizing insulin therapy in a diabetic rat model. J Periodontol 76:621–626
50. Siqueira JT, Cavalher-Machado SC, Arana-Chavez VE, Sannomiya P (2003) Bone formation around titanium implants in the rat tibia: role of insulin. Implant Dent 12:242–251
51. McCracken MS, Aponte-Wesson R, Chavali R, Lemons JE (2006) Bone associated with implants in diabetic and insulin treated rats. Clin Oral Implants Res 17:495–500
52. McCracken MS, Lemons JE, Rahemtulla F, Prince CW, Feldman D (2000) Bone response to titanium alloy implants placed in diabetic rats. Int J Oral Maxillofac Implants 15:345–354
53. Hasegawa H, Ozawa S, Hashimoto K, Takeichi T, Ogawa T (2008) Type 2 diabetes impairs implant osseointegration capacity in rats. Int J Oral Maxillofac Implants 23:237–246
54. Casap N, Nimri S, Ziv E, Sela J, Samuni Y (2008) Type 2 diabetes has minimal effect on osseointegration of titanium implants in *Psammomus obesus*. Clin Oral Implants Res 19:458–464
55. Kotsovilis S, Karoussis IK, Fourmousis I (2006) A comprehensive and critical review of dental implant placement in diabetic animals and patients. Clin Oral Implants Res 17:587–599
56. Lindhe J, Meyle J (2008) Group D of European workshop on periodontology. Peri-implant diseases: consensus report of the sixth European workshop on periodontology. J Clin Periodontol 35(8 suppl):282–285
57. Tawil G, Younan R, Azar P, Sleilati G (2008) Conventional and advanced implant treatment in the type II diabetic patient: surgical protocol and long-term clinical results. Int J Oral Maxillofac Implants 23:744–752
58. Meerwaldt R, Links T, Zeebregts C, Tio R, Hillebrands JL, Smit A (2008) The clinical relevance of assessing advanced glycation endproducts accumulation in diabetes. Cardiovasc Diabetol 7:29
59. Ulrich P, Cerami A (2001) Protein glycation, diabetes, and aging. Recent Prog Horm Res 56:1–21
60. Gangoiti MV, Cortizo AM, Arnol V, Felice JI, McCarthy AD (2008) Opposing effects of biphosphonates and advanced glycation end-products on osteoblastic cells. Eur J Pharmacol 600:140–147
61. McCarthy AD, Etcheverry SB, Bruzzone L, Lettieri G, Barrio DA, Cortizo AM (2001) Non-enzymatic glycosylation of a type I collagen matrix: effects on osteoblastic development and oxidative stress. BMC Cell Biol 2:16
62. McCarthy AD, Etcheverry SB, Bruzzone L, Cortizo AM (1997) Effects of advanced glycation end-products on the proliferation and differentiation of osteoblast-like cells. Mol Cell Biochem 170:43–51
63. Franke S, Siggelkow H, Wolf G, Hein G (2007) Advanced glycation endproducts influence the mRNA expression of RAGE, RANKL and various osteoblastic genes in human osteoblasts. Arch Physiol Biochem 113:154–161
64. Cortizo AM, Lettieri MG, Barrio DA, Mercer N, Etcheverry SB, McCarthy AD (2003) Advanced glycation end-products (AGEs) induce concerted changes in the osteoblastic expression of their receptor RAGE and in the activation of extracellular signal-regulated kinases (ERK). Mol Cell Biochem 250:1–10
65. McCarthy AD, Etcheverry SB, Cortizo AM (1999) Advanced glycation endproduct-specific receptors in rat and mouse osteoblast-like cells: regulation with stages of differentiation. Acta Diabetol 36:45–52
66. Schurman L, McCarthy AD, Sedlinsky C, Gangoiti MV, Arnol V, Bruzzone L, Cortizo AM (2008) Metformin reverts deleterious effects of advanced glycation end-products (AGEs) on osteoblastic cells. Exp Clin Endocrinol Diabetes 116:333–340

Chapter 6
Cannabinoids in Bone Repair

Itai A. Bab

Abbreviations

2-AG	2-Arachidonoylglycerol
β2AR	β2-Adrenergic receptors
BMP	Bone morphogenetic protein
DAGL	Diacylglycerol lipase
FAAH	Fatty acid amide hydrolase
IL-6	Interleukin 6
MAPK	Mitogen-activated protein kinase
M-CSF	Macrophage colony-stimulating factor
NAPE-PLD	*N*-acyl phosphatidylethanolamine phospholipase D
OGP	Osteogenic growth peptide
OPG	Osteoprotegerin
OVX	Ovariectomy
PTH	Parathyroid hormone
RANKL	Receptor activator of NFκB ligand
SNP	Single nucleotide polymorphism
THC	Δ9-Tetrahydrocannabinol
TRPV1	Transient receptor potential vanilloid type 1 receptor

The Marijuana plant, *Cannabis sativa*, has been cultivated throughout history for medical and recreational use. Its psychoactive properties are exploited generally for drug abuse. However, it is well established that in addition to its effect on the nervous system, it is involved in the functioning of other organs in the body.

I.A. Bab (✉)
Bone Laboratory, Institute of Dental Sciences,
The Hebrew University of Jerusalem, P.O. Box 12272, Jerusalem 91120, Israel
e-mail: babi@cc.huji.ac.il

J.J. Sela and I.A. Bab (eds.), *Principles of Bone Regeneration*,
DOI 10.1007/978-1-4614-2059-0_6, © Springer Science+Business Media, LLC 2012

The psychoactive component of marijuana and hashish, Δ9-tetrahydrocannabinol (THC), acts on two distinct receptors that are distributed throughout the body, only one of which mediates the psychotropic effects. These receptors respond to endogenous ligands, termed endocannabinoids, with THC just mimicking the activity of these physiological activators. The endocannabinoids are produced and degraded by specific enzymes. Together, the receptors, ligands, and enzymes comprise the endocannabinoid system. It is well established that THC produces numerous beneficial effects, including analgesia, appetite stimulation, nausea reduction, and reduction of intraocular pressure. THC also affects fertility, short-term memory, tumor growth, and motor coordination. Recently, there has been a rapidly growing interest in the role of cannabinoids in the regulation of skeletal remodeling and bone mass, addressed in basic, translational, and clinical research [1–13]. Studies published in the past decade propose an important role for the endocannabinoid system in the regulation of skeletal remodeling. The primarily neural CB1 cannabinoid receptor has been identified in sympathetic terminals innervating the skeleton. However, its function in controlling bone turnover is only partially understood. The predominantly peripheral CB2 receptor is expressed in bone cells. Its mechanism of action in bone cells, corroborated by human genetic considerations, has been reported in detail. Important genetic risk factors for low bone mass are attributed to polymorphism in CNR2, the gene encoding CB2. In this chapter, these considerations are extrapolated to address the potential role of the endocannabinoid system in bone wound healing. Several key components of the endocannabinoid system have been identified in bone. The main physiologic involvement of CB2 is associated with the maintenance of the balance of bone remodeling (Fig. 6.1). CB2 agonists are possible candidates for a combined anti-resorptive and anabolic therapy for osteoporosis. These considerations open an important therapeutic avenue in the treatment of impaired bone remodeling, bone healing, and bone implant acceptance, and control of bone mass and biomechanical function.

6.1 Cannabinoid Receptors and Ligands

CB1 and CB2 are G protein-coupled receptors [14], which share 44% of the overall identity (68% identity for the transmembrane domains). CB1 is perhaps the most abundantly expressed G protein-coupled receptor in the central nervous system. It is also present in peripheral neurons and gonads and to some extent in several other peripheral tissues. CB2 is expressed in the skeleton, immune system, cirrhotic liver, arteriosclerotic plaques, inflamed gastrointestinal mucosa, and glial and inflammatory cells in pathological brain conditions [15, 16]. That CB1 and CB2 are not functionally identical is demonstrated by the presence of cannabinoid agonists and antagonist with distinct binding specificities to either receptor [14–25]. Both receptors signal via the Gi/o subclass of G proteins, inhibiting stimulated adenylyl cyclase activity. Further downstream, the CBs induce the activation of p42/44 mitogen-activated protein kinase (MAPK), p38 MAPK, c-Jun N-terminal kinase, AP-1, the

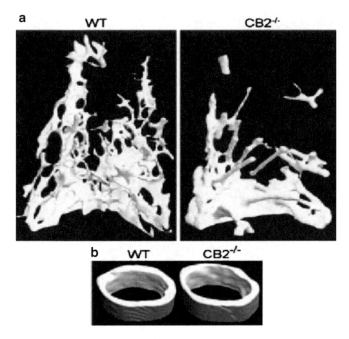

Fig. 6.1 Sever osteoporosis in femoral bones of aging CB2-deficient mice compared to wild-type (WT) femoral bones. Microcomputed tomographic images of trabecular bone in distal metaphysic (**a**) and mid-diaphysis (**b**)

neural form of focal adhesion kinase, protein kinase B, and K^+ and Ca^{2+} transients. Recently, it has been shown that the mitogenic action of CB2 in osteoblasts is mediated through a Gi-protein–Erk1/2–Mapkapk2–CREB–cyclin D1 axis (Fig. 6.2).

It has been proposed that GPR55 and TRPV1 may be also involved in endocannabinoid triggering of these event [26–34].

The main CB1 and CB2 endogenous ligands are N-arachidonoylethanolamide (AEA or anandamide) and 2-arachidonoylglycerol (2-AG). Anandamide is present in a variety of tissues such as the brain, kidney, liver, spleen, testis, uterus, and blood in picomol/g concentrations, with the highest levels reported in the central nervous system. The low anandamide concentrations have been attributed to low substrate levels and/or the short anandamide half-life in vivo. Anandamide is biosynthesized through N-acyl phosphatidylethanolamine phospholipase D (NAPE-PLD)-dependent and -independent pathways. The main anandamide degrading enzyme is fatty acid amide hydrolase (FAAH) [35–38]. In general, the tissue distribution of 2-AG is similar to that of anandamide. However, its concentration is three orders of magnitude higher (ng/g range). 2-AG production has been demonstrated in the central nervous system, platelets, and macrophages, especially in response to stimulation by inflammatory agents such as lipopolysaccharide. It is generated from arachidonic acid-enriched membrane phospholipids, such as inositol phospholipids, through the combined actions of phospholipase C and diacylglycerol lipases (DAGLα and DAGLβ). It is metabolized by a monoacylglycerol lipase (MAGL) [39–43].

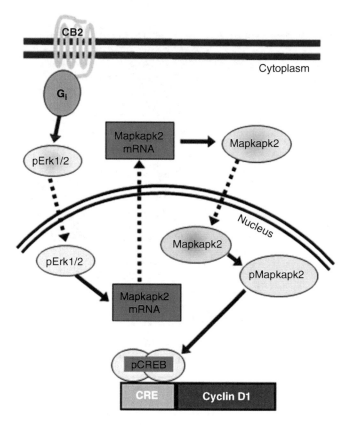

Fig. 6.2 Model of CB2 mitogenic signaling in osteoblasts

6.2 The Skeletal Endocannabinoid System

The major key components of the endocannabinoid system have been identified in bone (Fig. 6.3). Anandamide and 2-AG are present in this tissue at levels similar to those found in the brain. Because the blood endocannabinoid levels are several orders of magnitude lower than those found in bone, it is very likely that anandamide and 2-AG are synthesized locally in the skeleton. Indeed, both ligands are produced by osteoblasts and osteoclasts in culture. In addition, DAGLα and β are expressed in osteoblasts, osteocytes, and bone-lining cells (Fig. 6.4).

NAPE-PLD and FAAH are also expressed in bone cells. Although both 2-AG and anandamide are perceived as nonselective agonists of CB1 and CB2, findings in bone and bone cell cultures suggest differential effects of these ligands. While 2-AG activates CB1 in the sympathetic nerve terminals following a single or chronic administration to mice, thus stimulating bone formation, it has no effect on osteoblasts and may even act as an inverse agonist in these cells [16]. Like the CB2 selective

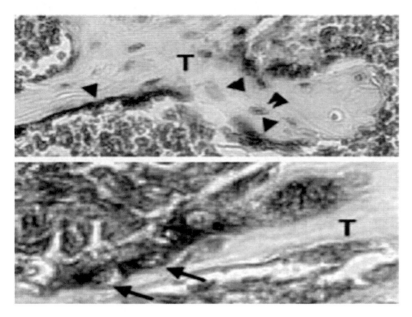

Fig. 6.3 Expression of CB2 in mouse osteoblasts, osteocytes, and osteoclast. T, trabecule; *arrows*, osteoclasts; *arrowheads*, osteoblasts; *double arrowheads*, osteocytes. Immunohistochemical staining using anti-CB2 antibodies

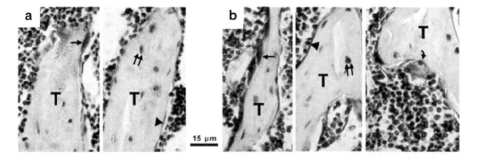

Fig. 6.4 Expression diacylglycerol lipase (DAGL) in bone cell. (**a**) DAGLα; (**b**) DAGLβ. T, bone trabecule; *arrows*, osteoblasts; *double arrows*, osteocytes; *arrow heads*, lining cells; *bent arrow*, osteoclasts

agonist, anandamide stimulates in vitro osteoblast proliferation. In addition, the number of osteoclasts in culture is increased by a direct challenge with anandamide or through the action of the FAAH inhibitor URB597 that leads to increased anandamide levels endogenously [15]. It remains to be seen whether these actions of anandamide are mediated by CB1, CB2, GPR55, and/or TRPV1.

6.3   Effects on Bone Cell Differentiation and Activity

Activation of CB2 has different effects in early osteoblast progenitors and in more mature osteoblastic cells. In the early precursors, represented by bone marrow-derived, partially differentiated osteoblastic cells that show limited CB2 expression, the specific CB2 agonist HU-308 [44] (Fig. 6.5), but not the specific CB1 agonist noladin ether [45], triggers a mitogenic effect and consequent expansion of the preosteo-blastic pool. Ex vivo osteoblastic colony (CFU-Ob) formation by bone marrow stromal cb2−/− cells is markedly diminished, whereas CFU-Ob formation by wild-type cells is stimulated by HU-308. In mature osteoblastic cells, represented by the MC3T3 E1 cell line, the same ligand stimulates osteoblast-differentiated functions such as alkaline phosphatase activity and matrix mineralization [13, 45]. Hence, CB2 signaling is involved in several regulatory, pro-osteogenic processes along the osteoblast lineage.

In mouse bone marrow-derived osteoclastogenic cultures, CB2 activation inhibits osteoclast formation by restraining mitogenesis at the monocytic stage, before incubation with RANKL. It also suppresses osteoclast formation by repressing RANKL expression in osteoblasts and osteoblast progenitors [40]. Likewise, it has been recently shown that the cannabinoid receptor agonist ajulemic acid also suppresses osteoclastogenesis [42]. By contrast, another study reported the stimulation of osteoclast formation and bone resorption by cannabinoid receptor agonists and their inhibition by antagonists [13, 44]. These allegedly paradoxical effects may be species and/or agonist dependent, as in human osteoclasts and other cells anandamide

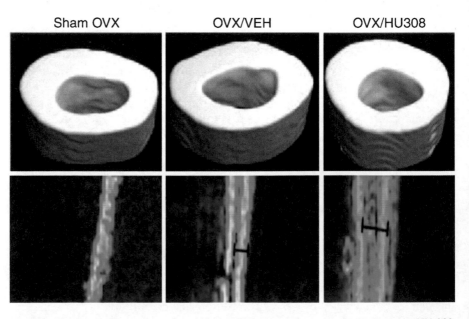

Fig. 6.5 Increased endosteal bone formation in OVX mice treated with the CB2 agonist HU-308

has been shown to activate also TRPV1. TRPV1 activation in the human osteoclasts and osteoclast precursors enhances osteoclast formation and activity and may modify the effect of selective CB2 agonists. In addition to CB2, low levels of CB1 mRNA have been reported in bone cell cultures [13, 44].

6.4   Skeletal Phenotypes of Cannabinoid Receptor-Deficient Mice

Cannabinoid receptor mutant mice have been used to assess the physiologic role of CB1 and CB2 in the control of bone mass. CB1-deficient mice have a low bone mass phenotype accompanied by increased osteoclast counts and decreased bone formation rate (Fig. 6.6). Our recent findings suggest that CB1 controls osteoblast function by negatively regulating norepinephrine (NE) release from sympathetic nerve terminals in the immediate vicinity of these cells.

NE suppresses bone formation by binding to osteoblastic β2AR [40]; this suppression is alleviated by activation of sympathetic CB1 (Fig. 6.7). That Cb1 agonists may be used to speed up bone wound healing is a corollary of the enhancement in fracture healing repeatedly reported in patients after traumatic brain injury (TBI) [45].

In a mouse model for TBI, we have demonstrated a critical regulatory role for CB1 and 2-AG in the stimulation of bone formation (Fig. 6.8). Therefore, peripherally selective specific CB1 agonists that do not cross the blood–brain barrier, and therefore do have any central adverse effects, could serve for the stimulation of

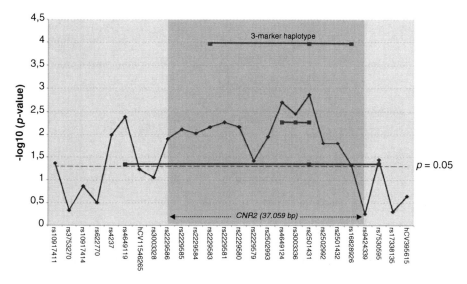

Fig. 6.6 Association of single nucleotide polymorphisms in the CNR2 gene with human osteoporosis

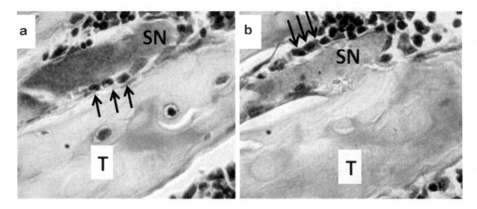

Fig. 6.7 CB1 expression in skeletal sympathetic nerve (SN) terminals. Serial sections stained with anti-tyrosine hydroxylases (**a**) and anti-CB1 (**b**) antibodies. T, trabecule; *arrows*, osteoblasts

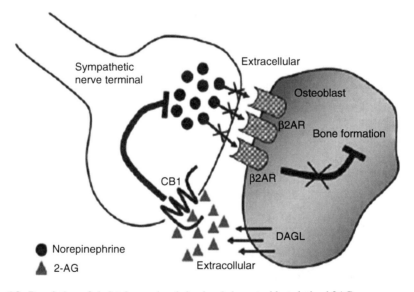

Fig. 6.8 Regulation of skeletal norepinephrine levels by osteoblast-derived 2AG

fracture repair. Alternatively, MAGL inhibitors could be used to stimulate CB1 by increasing the endogenous 2-AG levels. Animals with a CNR2-mutated gene have also a typical skeletal phenotype (Fig. 6.6). During their first 2–3 months of life, CNR2−/− mice accrue a normal peak trabecular bone mass, but later display a markedly enhanced age-related bone loss; their trabecular bone volume density at 1 year of age is approximately half compared to wild-type controls. Reminiscent of human postmenopausal osteoporosis, the CNR2−/− mice have a high bone turnover with increases in both bone resorption and formation which are at a net negative balance [38]. Importantly, low bone mass is the only spontaneous phenotype so far reported in these mice. Hence, because healthy CB2 mutant mice are otherwise normal, it appears that the main physiologic involvement of CB2 is associated with maintaining bone remodeling at balance. Polymorphisms in the human CNR1 and CNR2 loci were studied to assess the cannabinoid receptors as targets for the risk assessment and treatment of osteoporosis. The CNR1 locus is located on chromosome 5q15 and encompasses a single coding exon that is preceded by several noncoding 5′ exons, indicating a complex transcriptional regulation of this gene by different promoters. The CNR2 locus is located on chromosome 1p36. This genomic region and its mouse ortholog on chromosome 4 have been linked to BMD and osteoporosis in several independent association analyses. However, these analyses did not consider CNR2 as a potential candidate gene. Like CNR1, the CNR2 gene also consists of a single coding exon, which is preceded by a noncoding upstream exon. Thus far, two genetic association studies have been reported dealing with the relationship between polymorphisms in CNR genes and osteoporosis. The first study was carried out in a French Caucasian sample comparing postmenopausal osteoporotic women with a low bone mineral density (BMD) and age-matched healthy controls. Analysis of four single nucleotide polymorphisms (SNPs) spanning nearly 20 kb around the CB1 coding exon revealed no significant association with the osteoporosis phenotype, suggesting that the CNR1 locus does not have a major role in this sample. In the CNR2 gene, a total of 26 SNPs were analyzed, spanning approximately 300 kb around the CNR2 locus. Several of these SNPs showed a significant association with the disease phenotype, suggesting that CNR2 polymorphisms are important genetic risk factors for osteoporosis. The most significant p-values for allele and genotype associations were observed with SNPs located within the CB2 coding region ($p=0.0014$ and $p=0.00073$, respectively). Furthermore, when BMD at the lumbar spine was analyzed as a quantitative trait, highly significant differences were found in BMD between individuals carrying different SNPs in the CB2 coding region. Indeed, sequencing the CB2 coding exon in all patients and controls identified two missense variants, Gln63Arg and His316Tyr, with the Arg63 variant being more common in the osteoporotic patients than in the healthy controls. Taken together, these findings suggest that a common variant of the CB2 receptor contributes to the etiology of osteoporosis in humans. The second is a prospective study, which analyzed several candidate quantitative trait loci in BMD, including CNR2, in a cohort of 1,110 women and 1,128 Japanese men, 40–79 years of age [46]. For the *CNR2* locus, a single SNP (rs2501431, A→G) was assessed, which had shown the strongest association in the previously published French sample. BMD, measured by peripheral quantitative computed tomography or dual-energy X-ray absorptiometry, was consistently lower in women with the AA genotype compared to the AG and GG genotypes. Together, these studies strongly suggest that *CNR2* is the susceptibility gene for low BMD and osteoporosis on chromosome 1p36 [47–53].

References

1. Piomelli D (2003) The molecular logic of endocannabinoid signaling. Nat Rev Neurosci 4:873–884
2. Lambert DM, Fowler CJ (2005) The endocannabinoid system: drug targets, lead compounds, and potential therapeutic applications. J Med Chem 48:5059–5087
3. Hohmann AG, Suplita RL 2nd (2006) Endocannabinoid mechanisms of pain modulation. AAPS J 8:E693–E708
4. Pertwee RG (2006) Cannabinoid pharmacology: the first 66 years. Br J Pharmacol Suppl 1:S163–171
5. Kogan NM, Mechoulam R (2007) Cannabinoids in health and disease. Dialogues Clin Neurosci 9:413–430
6. Marx J (2006) Drug development. Drugs inspired by a drug. Science 311:322–325
7. Yazulla S (2008) Endocannabinoids in the retina: from marijuana to neuroprotection. Prog Retin Eye Res 27:501–526
8. Mechoulam R (2002) Discovery of endocannabinoids and some random thoughts on their possible roles in neuroprotection and aggression. Prostaglandins Leukot Essent Fatty Acids 66:93–99
9. Iversen L (2003) Cannabis and the brain. Brain 126:1252–1270
10. Akbas F, Gasteyger C, Sjodin A, Astrup A, Larsen TM (2009) A critical review of the cannabinoid receptor as a drug target for obesity management. Obes Rev 10:58–67
11. Bab I (2005) The skeleton: stone bones and stoned heads? In: Mechoulam R (ed) Cannabinoids as therapeutics, Milestones in drug therapy series. Birkhäuser, Basel, pp 201–206
12. Idris AI, Van 't Hof RJ, Greig IR, Ridge SA, Baker D, Ross RA et al (2005) Regulation of bone mass, bone loss and osteoclast activity by cannabinoid receptors. Nat Med 11:774–779
13. Howlett AC (2002) The cannabinoid receptors. Prostaglandins Other Lipid Mediat 68–69: 619–631
14. Julien B, Grenard P, Teixeira-Clerc F, Van Nhieu JT, Li L, Karsak M et al (2005) Antifibrogenic role of the cannabinoid receptor CB2 in the liver. Gastroenterology 128:742–755
15. Ledent C, Valverde O, Cossu G, Petitet F, Aubert JF, Beslot F et al (1999) Un responsiveness to cannabinoids and reduced addictive effects of opiates in CB1 receptor knockout mice. Science 283:401–404
16. Tam J, Ofek O, Fride E, Ledent C, Gabet Y, Müller R et al (2006) Involvement of neuronal cannabinoid receptor CB1 in regulation of bone mass and bone remodeling. Mol Pharmacol 70:786–792
17. Steffens S, Veillard NR, Arnaud C, Pelli G, Burger F, Staub C et al (2005) Low dose oral cannabinoid therapy reduces progression of atherosclerosis in mice. Nature 434:782–786
18. Shire D, Calandra B, Bouaboula M, Barth F, Rinaldi-Carmona M, Casellas P et al (1999) Cannabinoid receptor interactions with the antagonists SR 141716A and SR 144528. Life Sci 65:627–635
19. Hanus L, Breuer A, Tchilibon S, Shiloah S, Goldenberg D, Horowitz M et al (1999) HU-308: a specific agonist for CB(2), a peripheral cannabinoid receptor. Proc Natl Acad Sci USA 96:14228–14233
20. Howlett AC (2005) Cannabinoid receptor signaling. Handb Exp Pharmacol 53–79
21. Lauckner JE, Jensen JB, Chen HY, Lu HC, Hille B, Mackie K (2008) GPR55 is a cannabinoid receptor that increases intracellular calcium and inhibits M current. Proc Natl Acad Sci USA 105:2699–2704
22. Pertwee RG (2007) GPR55: a new member of the cannabinoid receptor clan? Br J Pharmacol 152:984–986
23. De Petrocellis L, Bisogno T, Maccarrone M, Davis JB, Finazzi-Agro A, Di Marzo V (2001) The activity of Anandamide at vanilloid VR1 receptors requires facilitated transport across the cell membrane and is limited by intracellular metabolism. J Biol Chem 276:12856–12863

24. Devane WA, Hanus L, Breuer A, Pertwee RG, Stevenson LA, Griffin G et al (1992) Isolation and structure of a brain constituent that binds to the cannabinoid receptor. Science 258: 1946–1949
25. Mechoulam R, Ben-Shabat S, Hanus L, Ligumsky M, Kaminski NE, Schatz AR et al (1995) Identification of an endogenous 2-monoglyceride, present in canine gut, that binds to cannabinoid receptors. Biochem Pharmacol 50:83–90
26. Willoughby KA, Moore SF, Martin BR, Ellis EF (1997) The biodisposition and metabolism of anandamide in mice. J Pharmacol Exp Ther 282:243–247
27. Simon GM, Cravatt BF (2006) Endocannabinoid biosynthesis proceeding through glycero-phospho-N-acyl ethanolamine and a role for alpha/beta-hydrolase 4 in this pathway. J Biol Chem 281:26465–26472
28. Cravatt BF, Demarest K, Patricelli MP, Bracey MH, Giang DK, Martin BR et al (2001) Super sensitivity to anandamide and enhanced endogenous cannabinoid signaling in mice lacking fatty acid amide hydrolase. Proc Natl Acad Sci USA 98:9371–9376
29. Varga K, Wagner JA, Bridgen DT, Kunos G (1998) Platelet- and macrophage-derived endog-enous cannabinoids are involved in endotoxin-induced hypotension. FASEB J 12:1035–1044
30. Di Marzo V, Bisogno T, De Petrocellis L, Melck D, Orlando P, Wagner JA et al (1999) Biosynthesis and inactivation of the endocannabinoid 2-arachidonoylglycerol in circulating and tumoral macrophages. Eur J Biochem 264:258–267
31. Stella N, Schweitzer P, Piomelli D (1997) A second endogenous cannabinoid that modulates long-term potentiation. Nature 388:773–778
32. Bisogno T, Howell F, Williams G, Minassi A, Cascio MG, Ligresti A et al (2003) Cloning of the first sn1-DAG lipases points to the spatial and temporal regulation of endocannabinoid signaling in the brain. J Cell Biol 163:463–468
33. Di Marzo V, Goparaju SK, Wang L, Liu J, Bátkai S, Járai Z et al (2001) Leptin-regulated endocannabinoids are involved in maintaining food intake. Nature 410:822–825
34. Panikashvili D, Simeonidou C, Ben-Shabat S, Hanus L, Breuer A, Mechoulam R et al (2001) An endogenous cannabinoid (2-AG) is neuroprotective after brain injury. Nature 413:527–531
35. Bab I, Ofek O, Tam J, Rehnelt J, Zimmer A (2008) Endocannabinoids and the regulation of bone metabolism. J Neuroendocrinol 20(Suppl 1):69–74
36. Tam J, Trembovler V, Di Marzo V, Petrosino S, Leo G, Alexandrovich A et al (2008) The can-nabinoid CB1 receptor regulates bone formation by modulating adrenergic signaling. FASEB J 22:285–294
37. Rossi F, Siniscalco D, Luongo L, De Petrocellis L, Bellini G, Petrosino S et al (2009) The endovanilloid/endocannabinoid system in human osteoclasts: possible involvement in bone formation and resorption. Bone 44:476–484
38. Bab I, Zimmer A (2008) Cannabinoid receptors and the regulation of bone mass. Br J Pharmacol 153:182–188
39. Hanus L, Abu-Lafi S, Fride E, Breuer A, Vogel Z, Shalev DE et al (2001) 2-arachidonyl glyc-eryl ether, an endogenous agonist of the cannabinoid CB1 receptor. Proc Natl Acad Sci USA 98:3662–3665
40. Ofek O, Karsak M, Leclerc N, Fogel M, Frenkel B, Wright K et al (2006) Peripheral cannabi-noid receptor, CB2, regulates bone mass. Proc Natl Acad Sci USA 103:696–701
41. Scutt A, Williamson EM (2007) Cannabinoids stimulate fibroblastic colony formation by bone marrow cells indirectly via CB2 receptors. Calcif Tissue Int 80:50–59
42. George KL, Saltman LH, Stein GS, Lian JB, Zurier RB (2008) Ajulemic acid, a non psychoac-tive cannabinoid acid, suppresses osteoclastogenesis in mononuclear precursor cells and induces apoptosis in mature osteoclast-like cells. J Cell Physiol 214:714–720
43. Idris AI, Sophocleous A, Landao-Bassonga E, Van 't Hof RJ, Ralston SH (2008) Regulation of bone mass, osteoclast function, and ovariectomy-induced bone loss by the type 2 cannabinoid receptor. Endocrinology 149:5619–5626
44. Bab I, Mechoulam R (2010) Oleoyl serine, an endogenous N-acyl amide, modulates bone remodeling and mass. Proc Natl Acad Sci USA 107:17710–17715

45. Amor S, Smith PA, Hart B, Baker D (2005) Biozzi mice: of mice and human neurological diseases. J Neuroimmunol 165:1–10
46. Yamada Y, Ando F, Shimokata H (2007) Association of candidate gene polymorphisms with bone mineral density in community-dwelling Japanese women and men. Int J Mol Med 19:791–801
47. Zimmer A, Zimmer AM, Hohmann AG, Herkenham M, Bonner TI (1999) Increased mortality, hypo activity, and hypoalgesia in cannabinoid CB1 receptor knockout mice. Proc Natl Acad Sci USA 96:5780–5785
48. McCaw E, Hu H, Gomez GT, Hebb AL, Kelly ME (2004) Denovan-Wright, EM. Structure, expression and regulation of the cannabinoid receptor gene (CB1) in Huntington's disease transgenic mice. Eur J Biochem 271:4909–4920
49. Brown JP, Delmas PD, Malaval L, Edouard C, Chapuy MC, Meunier PJ (1984) Serum bone Gla-protein: a specific marker for bone formation in postmenopausal osteoporosis. Lancet 1: 1091–1093
50. Nogueira-Filho Gda R, Cadide T, Rosa BT, Neiva TG, Tunes R, Peruzzo D, Nociti FH Jr, César-Neto JB (2008) Cannabis sativa smoke inhalation decreases bone filling around titanium implants: a histomorphometric study in rats. Implant Dent 17:461–470
51. Zhang P, Ishiguro H, Ohtsuki T, Hess J, Carillo F, Walther D et al (2004) Human cannabinoid receptor 1: 5' exons, candidate regulatory regions, polymorphisms, haplotypes and association with polysubstance abuse. Mol Psychiatry 9:916–931
52. Devoto M, Shimoya K, Caminis J, Ott J, Tenenhouse A, Whyt MP et al (1998) First-stage autosomal genome screen in extended pedigrees suggests genes predisposing to low bone mineral density on chromosomes 1p, 2p and 4q. Eur J Hum Genet 6:151–157
53. Karsak M, Cohen-Solal M, Freudenberg J, Ostertag A, Morieux C, Kornak U et al (2005) Cannabinoid receptor type 2 gene is associated with human osteoporosis. Hum Mol Genet 14:3389–3396

Part III
Bridging of Skeletal Defects and Implants

Chapter 7
Mesenchymal Stem Cells for Bone Gene Therapy

Gadi Pelled, Olga Mizrahi, Nadav Kimelman-Bleich, and Dan Gazit

Bone tissue has regenerative capabilities enabling the self-repair and regeneration of fractures and other forms of damage. However, in extreme situations where the extent of bone loss or damage due to trauma, surgery, or metabolic diseases such as osteoporosis is too large, full regeneration will not occur. In these situations, the extent of bone loss, or the conditions leading to its loss, is beyond the capabilities of the bone self-repair mechanism. Large bone defects that do not spontaneously heal are thus called nonunion defects, and they present a major problem for orthopedic surgeons. Currently, nonunion fractures are treated by metallic implants that tend to fail in the long run. In addition, extensive bone formation is required in spine surgery when a fusion of two vertebrae is considered in the treatment for intervertebral disc degeneration leading to back pain. It is clear, therefore, that for these clinical conditions a biological approach that will be able to enhance bone formation is required. Most of the biological approaches undertaken to overcome the loss of large bone segments involve the administration of either cells with osteogenic potential or of osteogenic growth factors. Both approaches are aimed at enhancing the bone formation process by introducing one of its components: i.e., bone forming cells and osteogenic growth factors that promote the proliferation and differentiation of osteoprogenitors into mature osteoblasts that are responsible for the lay-down of new bone tissue. Gene therapy was applied to this setting as a means to deliver recombinant DNA sequences encoding for the osteogenic growth factors. However, in delivering the desired gene in vivo, two strategies may be taken:

1. The direct delivery of the construct via viral or nonviral vectors or
2. The delivery of the desired gene product via cells that were genetically engineered to express the desired gene, ex vivo. The latter approach is termed Cell-Based Gene Therapy, and it will be the main focus of this chapter.

G. Pelled (✉) • O. Mizrahi, MSc • N. Kimelman-Bleich • D. Gazit
Department of Surgery and Cedars-Sinai Regenerative Medicine Institute (CS-RMI),
Cedars-Sinai Medical Center, Los Angeles, California, USA
e-mail: gadip@ekmd.huji.ac.il; olga.golzand@mail.huji.ac.il;
  nadavk@ekmd.huji.ac.il; dgaz@cc.huji.ac.il

J.J. Sela and I.A. Bab (eds.), *Principles of Bone Regeneration*,
DOI 10.1007/978-1-4614-2059-0_7, © Springer Science+Business Media, LLC 2012

7.1 Stem Cells

Stem cells are a distinct population of cells that can give rise to different tissues. Two main features characterize all types of stem cells: self-renewal and the ability to give rise to differentiating daughter cells. Stem cells can be further divided into two major groups. The first group constitutes the embryonic stem (ES) cells, which together with the totipotent zygote present a cell population able to develop into a multitude of cell types and tissues [1]. The second group constitutes adult stem cells, which reside in adult tissues and give rise to differentiated, tissue-specialized cells. These adult stem cells are responsible for the regenerative capacities of tissues in the body. Generally, adult stem cells present a more limited range of differentiation compared with ES cells. In studies done by Jiang et al., it was reported that multipotent adult progenitor cells (MAPCs) purified from adult bone marrow can differentiate at the single cell level, to cells with visceral mesoderm, neuroectoderm, and endoderm characteristics in vitro [2]. Adult stem cells are preferable for therapeutic purposes since they are considered safer for transplantation with lesser proliferation capacity and tumorogenecity than ES cells. In addition, adult stem cells are more easily directed to specific lineages than ES cells which can give rise to a wide range of tissues following local transplantation [3]. Skeletal tissues such as bone, cartilage, tendon, and ligament that are the focus of orthopedic medicine vary in their ability to self-regenerate. While bone tissue is considered to have high regeneration capacity and ligament tissue a somewhat lesser degree, cartilage tissue is considered to have a very low self-repair ability [4, 5]. All these tissues are believed to have originated from similar common stem cells termed mesenchymal stem cells (MSCs). MSCs are stem cells residing in a variety of adult mesenchymal tissues. The MSCs and their self-repair ability correlate with their capability in recruitment of adult MSCs from their local environment [6, 7].

MSCs were readily isolated from the bone marrow and expanded in culture [8]. They were shown to differentiate into various mesenchymal lineages including bone, cartilage, adipose, muscle, and tendon [9]. Their accessibility and ease to manipulate in vitro have made them natural candidates for orthopedic gene therapy studies and the focus for the development of therapeutic approaches in orthopedic therapy. However, bone marrow-derived MSCs are not the only stem cells found to differentiate to various skeletal tissues. Stem cells from other tissues, such as muscle and adipose tissue, were also found to have similar properties [10, 11].

7.2 Bone Marrow-Derived MSCs for Bone Gene Therapy

Since MSCs and osteoprogenitors are relatively easily isolated from bone marrow and cultured in vitro, it is conceivable to use them as vehicles for the delivery of therapeutic genes in vivo, a strategy known as stem cell-based gene therapy [12]. Most gene therapy studies directed to bone healing attempt to induce bone formation in a model of bone nonunion fractures or as a means to achieve spinal fusion.

Indeed, some studies have used primary MSCs and cell lines for the expression and delivery of osteogenic genes inducing bone formation [13–17]. These studies implemented various types of MSCs including cell lines such as C3H10T1/2 and primary marrow-derived stem cells for the delivery of bone morphogenetic protein-2 (BMP-2). The delivery of growth factors of the bone morphogenetic protein family is often used in these studies, since these factors promote osteogenic differentiation and bone formation [18, 19]. In particular, BMP-2 was commonly used because it is a highly osteoinductive agent, well studied and known to induce bone in vivo in ectopic and orthotropic sites [18, 20–30]. Other members of the BMP family, such as BMP-4 and -9, were also used for stem cell-mediated gene therapy [31–36]. The hypothesis of these studies was that healing of bone defects could be achieved by long-term production of osteoinductive agents in the vicinity of bone defects, inducing new bone formation and defect repair.

Bone marrow-derived MSCs are good candidates for gene therapy directed to bone regeneration, not only because of their accessibility, but also because they form the source stem cells for osteoprogenitors and osteoblasts, the bone forming cells, in the bone environment [6]. Osteogenic differentiation begins with the commitment of the undifferentiated MSC to the osteogenic lineage, giving rise to committed osteoprogenitor cells that gradually differentiate into mature osteoblasts [6]. It was postulated that using genetically engineered MSCs for bone cell-mediated gene therapy may have a particular advantage [12]. When these cells are engineered to express osteogenic growth factors such as BMP-2, upon transplantation in vivo, the expressed transgene exerts its effect not only on host mesenchymal tissue (paracrine effect) but also on the engineered MSCs (autocrine effect). Thus, the engrafted, engineered MSCs differentiate and contribute to the bone formation process and in parallel recruit and induce osteogenic differentiation in other host stem cells (Fig. 7.1). It was hypothesized that these dual autocrine and paracrine effects may promote bone formation to a larger extent than any other cell type merely exerting a paracrine effect. Using murine C3H10T1/2 MSC line that were engineered to express BMP-2, the authors were able to demonstrate their increased osteogenic potential over non-MSCs engineered CHO cell lines that also expressed BMP-2 [12]. Engineered MSCs were able to heal murine nonunion radial defects to a greater extent than non-osteogenic CHO cells, despite the fact that these cells secreted more BMP-2 protein than the engineered MSCs.

Using MSCs as vehicles for gene delivery has an additional benefit over direct in vivo delivery of proteins or genes. Engineered MSCs can potentially engraft into the damaged tissue in vivo and express the therapeutic genes for long periods, whereas local, one time administration of genes or protein will have a limited time effect. BMP family members are known for their ability to induce bone formation in vivo and repair bone defects when applied locally in the injury sites [37–39]. In order to compare the efficiency of stem cell-mediated gene therapy with BMP-2 protein delivery, Moutsatsos et al. have analyzed the extent of bone tissue produced by engineered MSCs (C3H10T1/2) expressing BMP-2 compared with local administration of a high dose of BMP-2 in a murine radial nonunion defect [40].

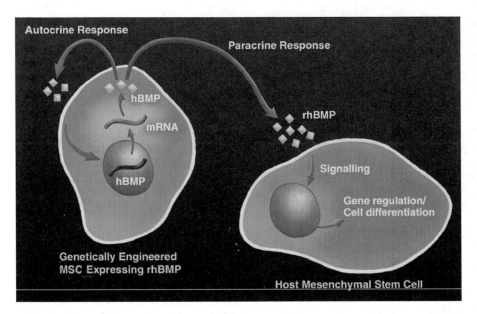

Fig. 7.1 Genetically engineered MSCs exert both autocrine and paracrine responses leading to a synergistic effect of osteogenesis in vivo

The authors have found that the engineered MSCs produced significantly more bone tissue then was produced following local administration of BMP-2 protein.

MSCs or osteoprogenitor cell-mediated gene therapy holds yet another advantage over protein delivery or even other types of gene delivery. When analyzing the healing process in bone defects following transplantation of MSCs engineered to express rhBMP-2, an interesting pattern is observed. Engineered MSCs have produced bone in an organized manner by augmenting new bone on top of the defect edges, forming continuous regeneration between the original defect edges and the newly formed bone [12, 40, 41]. In comparison, BMP-2 protein delivery or the implantation of non-MSCs CHO cells expressing BMP-2 resulted in the formation of diffused bone foci with no continuity to the original bone [12]. This phenomenon can be attributed to the ability of MSCs to localize and orient themselves to particular sites in the defect area following transplantation. It was found that MSCs localized mainly surrounding the defect edges rather than being randomly distributed in the defect site [12]. Apparently, being stem cells, MSCs can respond to local factors and developmental signals that direct and guide their orientation in the transplantation site and affect the healing process in a manner similar to the process that takes place during bone formation in developmental stages. Liechty et al. demonstrated that human MSCs possessed these characteristics by showing that these cells were able to engraft in various fetal mesenchymal tissues following systemic administration in utero in sheep [9]. Moreover, human MSCs were able to localize into the osteoprogenitor layers of calvaria bone when transplanted subcutaneously adjacent to the calvaria in SCID mice [42].

Human bone marrow-derived MSCs are expected to have the same regenerative benefits described above for murine MSCs. However, if stem cells engraft and respond to local signals, what possible advantage does genetic engineering have? This question is stressed in the case of human MSCs which were previously found to regenerate bone in vivo upon local transplantation to bone defect, even without any genetic engineering [43]. On the other hand, additional studies have shown that human MSCs cannot form bone when engineered to express the LacZ gene or nonengineered at all, compared with human MSCs engineered to express BMP-2 [41]. It was found that human MSCs infected with adenoviral vector encoding for human BMP-2 were able to differentiate to osteogenic cells both in vitro and in vivo forming cartilage and bone tissues, and healing nonunion defects created in CD nude mice [29, 41]. Human MSCs infected with adenoviral vector encoding the LacZ reporter gene were not able to form bone or cartilage in vivo. The type of matrix used to carry for human cells when delivered in vivo could explain this discrepancy. It was found that the ability of human MSCs to form bone in vivo is dependent upon osteoinductive matrices such as hydroxyapatite/TCP that are non-biodegradable [44]. Consequently, genetic engineering of human MSCs may elicit the osteogenic potential of MSCs regardless of the carrier type with the use of biodegradable carriers [41, 45]. One can safely assume that in large bone defects, nonengineered human MSCs will not be sufficient in order to induce repair compared to genetically engineered cells. The above-mentioned studies demonstrate the unique features that MSCs possess, granting them additional advantage for the use in bone gene therapy and gene delivery. These stem cells can serve as "smart" vehicles that in addition to expressing the transgene in specific areas of the damaged tissue can also actively participate in the neo-tissue formation process.

7.3   Cell Sources for Stem Cell-Mediated Bone Gene Therapy

Adult MSCs that reside in the bone marrow are the natural stem cells for bone forming cells, since this is the natural reservoir from which cells are recruited for bone repair. However, this does not exclude the use of other sources of stem cells for bone gene therapy. The most prominent cells studied in this regard are fat and muscle stem cells [11, 46–52]. Muscle-derived stem cells can be conveniently isolated from a muscle biopsy and expanded in vitro. Muscle tissue contains stem cells with the ability to differentiate into osteoblasts under the influence of a proper osteogenic factor such as BMP-2 [10]. These cells though originating from murine muscle tissue, following engineering to express BMP-2 or BMP-4, were able to differentiate into osteoblasts and osteocytes and could heal critical nonunion bone defects in the calvaria [50, 53]. Likewise, engineered cells from human skeletal muscle were shown to have in vitro and in vivo osteogenic potential when engineered to express rhBMP-2 [49]. Since a muscle cell is one of the possible differentiation pathways of MSCs, these results are not surprising.

Fat tissue-derived stem cells can also respond to BMP signaling by converting from the adipogenic differentiation pathway toward the osteogenic one [47, 52, 54]. These stem cells could be obtained from routine liposuction procedures and cultured in vitro. Osteogenic differentiation of adipose-derived stem cells was induced by the over-expression of BMP-2 and was further used for the healing of critical sized femoral defects and induce spinal fusion [48, 51, 55]. MAPCs that were co-purified with MSCs from adult marrow differentiated not only into mesenchymal cells but also into cells with mesoderm, neuroectoderm, and endoderm characteristics in vitro. In vivo, MAPCs engrafted and differentiated to the hematopoietic lineage and to the epithelium of liver, lung, and gut. However, these cells were not integrated in skeletal tissues, an issue which might be attributed to the low turnover characteristic of these tissues [2]. Nevertheless, as MAPCs proliferate at a high rate, they may also be considered as another source for stem cell-mediated therapy. ES cells originating from the inner cell mass of an embryo in the blastocyst stage have a wide differentiation potential both in vitro and in vivo. These cells can give rise to a variety of cell types including neural cells, cardiomyocytes, vascular cells, and hematopoietic cells [56]. They were also found to differentiate into osteogenic cells in vitro [57, 58]. However, there is still no data on osteogenic differentiation in vivo. In addition, the method of obtaining human ES cells introduces some major ethical issues [59, 60]. Moreover, it was found that MAPCs obtained from the bone marrow possess a pluripotent range of differentiation that includes all cell types found in the embryo [61]. For these reasons, one can expect that ES cells will not be the main target cells for gene therapy applications in orthopedics in the future, whereas the more easily obtained, manipulated, and less controversial MSCs will be a more realistic choice.

7.4 Angiogenesis and Bone Gene Therapy

Most gene therapy strategies to facilitate bone regeneration, as was discussed above, focus on the delivery and expression of osteoinductive genes, such as members of the BMP family. Such growth factors promote osteogenic differentiation of MSCs, osteoprogenitors, and osteoblasts. This approach is aimed at initiating and promoting the primary process that is responsible for osteogenesis. A different, novel approach was suggested that targets initiating secondary processes supporting new bone formation by promoting angiogenesis [32, 40, 62]. Angiogenesis was found to be closely correlated to enchondral bone formation during development [40, 63]. It was found that vascular endothelial growth factor (VEGF), a known inducer of angiogenesis, couples the transition from cartilage to bone in developing bones. Moreover, it was found that applying TNP-470, an angiogenesis inhibitor, could markedly reduce BMP-2-induced ectopic bone formation in muscle tissue. Other studies have found a correlation between angiogenesis and GDF-5, a member of the BMP family, and SMAD5, a BMP signal molecule [64–66]. Moutsatsos et al. reported an important finding linking angiogenesis and together with new bone formation induced by BMP-2 secreting MSCs [40]. Increased blood vessel formation was observed, coupled with new bone and cartilage created in ectopic muscle tissue transplanted with engineered MSCs. A CAM assay further indicated that BMP-2 protein induced angiogenesis and may, in part, mediate the angiogenesis observed in transplants of genetically engineered MSCs in vivo [40]. These studies clearly indicate the important supporting effect that angiogenesis and its mediator, VEGF, have on bone formation.

The use of angiogenic growth factors for bone formation was demonstrated by Peng et al. In this study, the authors implemented a combination of BMP-4 and VEGF genes both infected into muscle-derived stem cells. It was found that VEGF alone expressed in muscle stem cells did not elicit any bone response; however, when expressed together with BMP-4, a synergistic effect of VEGF and BMP-4 was observed. Timing and ratio between VEGF and BMP-4 expression were found to be most crucial in this study [67]. Once again, the importance of angiogenesis in new bone formation was demonstrated when the soluble VEGF antagonist Flt1 was able to inhibit new bone formation elicited by BMP-4. These authors have also shown similar, but not identical, effects on accelerated bone formation when they combined BMP-2 and VEGF-expressing muscle-derived stem cells [67]. These studies represent a new approach, which combines two growth factors that promote key role processes in bone formation.

7.5   Gene Therapy for Systemic Bone Diseases

The most common pathology in bone that has been addressed by gene therapy studies was nonunion bone defects [12–16, 32, 40, 41, 45, 49, 50, 67]. As discussed above, adult stem cell-based gene therapy has successfully addressed this problem in animal models by using MSCs of bone marrow, adipose tissue or muscle origin, genetically engineered to express osteogenic growth factors, primarily members of the BMP family, which were transplanted in the fracture site. Several studies have aimed to develop gene therapy for systemic and metabolic bone diseases. These diseases present more complex pathologies since they require systemic rather than local repair and also the possible involvement of different genes.

Osteoporosis is a disease resulting in bone loss and osteopenia. Though the results of bone loss are the same, two types of osteoporosis are commonly recognized: Type I or postmenopausal osteoporosis and Type II or senile osteoporosis [68, 69]. Type I is related to increased osteoclastogenesis resulting in over resorption of bone due to estrogen depletion, whereas Type II is related to decreased osteogenesis due to bone marrow MSCs senescence, that is reflected by decreased number, proliferation, and osteogenic activity [70–74]. Although osteoclastogenesis is increased in Type I osteoporosis, there is ample evidence of decreased osteogenesis as well [75]. It is therefore a rational approach to attempt to increase bone mass in osteoporosis by increasing osteogenesis. Indeed, Turgeman et al. have shown that systemic administration of BMP-2 protein to osteoporotic mice of both Type I and Type II osteoporosis models has resulted in increased osteogenic potential of bone marrow MSCs leading to restoration of bone mass [70]. Moreover, the same group has shown that human bone marrow MSCs obtained from osteoporotic patients had increased osteogenic activity and proliferation following infection with adenoviral vector encoding for BMP-2 [41]. The engineered cells were able to form bone in vivo and regenerate nonunion defects in CD nude mice. These studies indicated the potential use of bone marrow MSCs engineered to express osteogenic growth factor as BMP-2 for the treatment of osteoporosis. Since bone marrow MSCs are affected in both Type I and Type II osteoporosis, it is conceivable to target these cells for gene therapy applications.

An opposite approach directed at blocking osteoclastogenesis was suggested by Goater et al. to prevent the loosening of prosthetic implants due to bone resorption. The authors engineered synovial fibroblasts to express osteoprotegrin (OPG), a RANKL receptor antagonist that counteracts the osteoclast differentiation action of RANKL [76]. Engineered fibroblasts were able to inhibit osteoclastogenesis induced by debris in mouse calvaria. This approach can be easily duplicated and applied to the bone marrow in osteoporosis using MSCs as vehicles for OPG expression. However, in this approach MSCs would serve merely as vehicles for OPG delivery and would not have an anabolic influence on bone formation. Another interesting approach directed mainly toward age-related bone loss due to Type I osteoporosis was suggested by Yudoh et al. The authors' approach was directed toward the pathological mechanism of senescence affecting bone marrow osteoblasts, which subsequently leads to low bone mass. In order to overcome this, the authors transduced human osteoblasts and osteoblastic cell lines that display senescence phenotype with the telomerase reverse transcriptase (hTERT) gene [77]. The forced expression of hTERT resulted in increased telomerase activity in these cells, and consequently elevated replication capacity and delayed senescence were observed. It was the authors' suggestion to further use this approach for cell-based gene therapy for osteoporosis. Osteopetrosis is a genetic disease that results in the opposite phenotype of osteoporosis. Excessive bone is formed, eliminating the bone marrow from the bone compartment and eventually resulting in death due to lack of sufficient hematopoiesis [78]. Osteopetrosis is caused by a decrease in osteoclastogenesis due to a genetic mutation of essential growth factors important for osteoclast development such as CSF-1. The op/op mouse carries a genetic defect in CSF-1 and serves as a model for osteopetrosis. Abboud et al. have suggested the over-expression of soluble forms of CSF-1, specifically in osteoblasts, as a potential model of gene therapy for osteopetrosis [79]. To corroborate the notion that expression of CSF-1 by osteoblasts can restore the osteopetrotic phenotype, the authors have created a transgenic op/op mouse that harbors the CSF-1 cDNA under the control of the osteoblastic-specific osteocalcin promoter. The authors report that within 5 weeks postnatal, the osteopetrotic phenotype was completely reversed to the wild-type phenotype. Bone marrow derived could be potentially transduced to express the CSF-1 gene, returned to the bone marrow and promote osteoclastogenesis.

Osteogenesis imperfecta is a genetic disease that affects the quality of the bone formed in the body. Due to a mutation in one of the subtypes of procollagen chain genes, the resulting assembly and production of mature collagen fibers are impaired [78]. In order to overcome this genetic mutation; the delivery of the correct form of collagen pro-chain gene must be achieved. The *oim* mouse model, which harbors a defect in Proα2(I)-chain gene, presents a phenotype resembling osteogenesis imperfecta. Niyibizi et al. have shown evidence for a potential therapeutic use of stem cell-based gene therapy in osteogenesis imperfecta. They have over-expressed the correct Proα2(I) cDNA in *oim* mice bone marrow-derived MSCs using an adenovirus. The authors reported that the corrected gene was expressed in vitro, and the cells were able to form a stable Type I collagen fiber composed of Proα1(I) and Proα2(I) in the correct ratio of 2:1 [80]. The studies mentioned above demonstrated that MSCs play a crucial role in the pathophysiology of systemic and metabolic bone diseases. However, even in cases where the pathophysiology is not directly connected to MSCs, they can still serve as powerful candidates for cell-mediated gene therapy.

7.6 Genetic Engineering of MSCs

The relative ease of MSC isolation from different skeletal tissues and expansion in vitro has made them readily available for genetic manipulation with various vectors. The most common vectors that have been used were adenoviral vectors [29, 41, 49, 50, 80]. Retroviral vectors have also been used for transducing MSCs and osteoprogenitors but with relatively poor results [15]. Modifications of retroviral infection techniques were suggested to improve the transduction rate of MSCs with these vectors. Kuhlcke et al. showed positive results when tissue culture vessels were preloaded with retroviral vectors by low-speed (1,000 g) centrifugation [81]. Various cell types cultured in these conditions were efficiently transduced into T cells with up to 85% efficiency. Recently, the use of a Lentiviral vector encoding for the BMP-2 gene has been shown to be effective in expressing the transgene in rat MSCs leading to osteogenesis in vitro and in vivo [82, 83]. MSCs were also effectively transduced with other vectors such as vesicular stomatitis virus (VSV) [84–86]. Human bone marrow-derived MSCs were found to be highly susceptible to VSV infection achieving high rates of transduction with more than 81% efficiency [84]. A safety aspect was also encountered as transduction with VSV did not alter the proliferation and differentiation potential of bone marrow-derived MSCs.

Achieving high transgene expression is a desired goal in some cases in gene therapy. An interesting and novel approach was undertaken by Peng et al. for enhancing the secretion of BMP-4 transgene from transduced bone marrow MSCs, ex vivo [87]. The authors used an MFG-based retroviral vector pseudotyped with a VSV-G envelope. In order to increase BMP-4 secretion, the authors created hybrid constructs encoding for BMP-4 peptide linked to a BMP-2 propeptide sequence. Replacement of the BMP-4 propeptide region with that of BMP-2 has resulted in increased secretion of BMP-4 from MSCs engineered to express this hybrid.

Achieving high expression of a transgene is not always the ultimate goal of stem cell-based gene therapy, especially in orthopedics. Limiting the expression in terms of intensity and duration is necessary in certain cases. One way to ensure limited expression of the transgene is the use of tissue-specific promoters. Bone- and osteoblast-specific promoters will ensure expression in the bone marrow zone where active synthesis of bone matrix occurs. Stover et al. used the collagen1A1 promoter sequence in order to achieve osteoblastic-specific expression [88]. Expression of a marker gene regulated by the tissue specific promoter was limited to osteoblasts both in vitro in MSC cultures and in vivo in chimeric embryos. A similar approach using the osteocalcin promoter was undertaken by Abboud et al. where osteoblasts were engineered to express CSF-1 for the treatment of osteopetrosis. Maintaining expression limited for osteoblasts is important to prevent the expression in other cell types and is more required in genetic skeletal diseases or systemic metabolic diseases such as osteopetrosis and osteoporosis. For local skeletal defects, this approach is less relevant, since the required transgene expression is limited to a short period of time, and the exact type of cells that expresses it is not critical for the repair. Fine-tuning of transgene expression and temporal control on the duration of expression may be critical in the future development of gene therapy applications for orthopedic medicine. The use of tetracycline-regulated promoters to manage transgene expression was suggested [17, 40]. Using a Tet-off promoter system in the MSC line, C3H10T1/2, where tetracycline presence inhibited BMP-2 transgene expression, it was shown that engineered MSCs expressed and secreted BMP-2 only in the absence of tetracycline. The presence of tetracycline in vitro and the addition of tetracycline to the drinking water of mice transplanted with these genetically engineered MSCs completely inhibited BMP-2 expression. In vitro, BMP-2 regulation by tetracycline has resulted in the control of the engineered MSCs osteogenic differentiation. In conditions promoting BMP-2 expression, osteogenic differentiation of engineered MSCs was induced. In contrast, this was not evident when the transgene was suppressed, i.e., in the presence of tetracycline. In in vivo experiments, where engineered MSCs were transplanted both ectopically in muscle tissue and in radial nonunion bone defect, it was found that bone formation and nonunion defect regeneration were both dependent on tetracycline control. Tetracycline administrated to mice transplanted with the engineered cells completely inhibited bone formation and defect regeneration otherwise observed when tetracycline was not administered. This study demonstrated the potential of exogenously regulated promoters. Such promoters have the potential to allow the control over the duration and intensity of transgene expression and therefore to modulate in real time its biological effect. Such constructs can be used in both chronic systemic and metabolic diseases, such as osteoporosis, that may need long-term gene expression and regulation, and for local injury and temporal disease. In the latter case, regulated constructs that will not integrate permanently to the cells are preferable.

7.7   Future Prospects

As is evident from the above-reviewed studies, MSCs present a great advantage for stem cell-mediated gene therapy directed for orthopedic medicine. MSCs can be isolated from various tissues, the most common of which are bone marrow, adipose, and muscle tissues. Although many studies on the immunoisolation based on surface markers of MSCs have been performed, the various selected MSC subtypes are indistinguishable [89]. Some evidence indicates that MSCs may even be retrieved from peripheral blood [89]. Together with molecular studies directed at finding distinct molecular markers of MSCs, future development may provide us with a reliable technique for purifying and expanding in vitro blood circulating MSCs, which are more easily retrieved.

Since most of the studies performed on nonunion defect models were highly successful, it is expected that large animal studies are to follow, possibly leading toward first clinical trials. It is expected that additional cell-meditated gene therapy studies involving other genes with osteogenic potential will be undertaken [90, 91]. As MSCs present a multi-lineage differentiation potential, further studies are expected to examine MSC advantages and relying on their ability to differentiate to various lineages for the regeneration of skeletal tissues. Investigations may evolve following other studies elucidating the signal transduction pathways of mesenchymal tissue differentiation and identifying novel genes that can trigger lineage-specific differentiation of MSCs.

The increasing understanding and recognition of the complexity of skeletal tissue formation has led to the discovery of mechanisms that support skeletal tissue development and/or regeneration. This has been exemplified by the discovery of the important role of angiogenesis in bone development and regeneration as discussed above. Moreover, this has addressed the complexity of bone regeneration and its mechanisms by expressing both BMP-4 and VEGF, and therefore achieving a synergistic effect between the two mechanisms of osteogenic differentiation and angiogenesis. Expressing several genes that are applied for different specific mechanisms in order to promote skeletal tissue development and regeneration should be in the scope of future gene therapy strategies applied for skeletal regeneration. Such complex approaches should also pave the way for the development of MSC-based therapeutic applications for systemic and metabolic bone diseases, like osteoporosis, which have several mechanisms involved in their pathophysiology.

A major hurdle to overcome in tissue engineering is an insufficient supply of oxygen to newly forming tissue. Insufficient oxygen results in cell death [92, 93] and loss or delay of cell differentiation [94], especially with regard to osteogenesis, which is dependent on vascularization and oxygen supply [95]. One option in overcoming hypoxic conditions within a tissue-engineering scaffold is to increase the level of oxygen within the scaffold by using perfluorocarbons (PFCs) such as PFTBA. PFCs have a linear relationship between oxygen partial pressure and oxygen concentration [96]. While oxygen solubility in water is only 2.2 mM, oxygen solubility in PFTBA is 35 mM, a 15- to 20-fold increase over solubility in water alone [97]. In a recent study, in which BMP2 expressing MSCs were implanted in ectopic and orthotropic sites in PFTBA supplemented fibrin gel, the positive effect of this material on bone formation was demonstrated. In the ectopic site, there were significant increases in bone formation (2.5-fold increase), cell survival, and *osteocalcin* activity in the PFTBA-supplemented groups. PFTBA supplementation significantly increased structural parameters of bone in radial bone defects and triggered a significant 1.4-fold increase in bone volume in the spinal fusion model. Synthetic oxygen carrier supplementation of tissue-engineered implants enhanced ectopic bone formation and yielded better bone quality and volume in bone repair and spinal fusion models, probably due to increased cell survival [98].

Finally, it is expected that engineered MSCs combined with specially designed polymeric scaffolds will soon be used for skeletal tissue engineering both in vivo and ex vivo. Combining MSCs with a particular growth factor gene that directs their differentiation and that triggers the process of tissue formation is a good approach to engineering tissues. Here as well, the properties of MSCs that enable them to differentiate and express growth factors can be exploited for the purposes of tissue engineering.

To conclude, MSCs as reviewed here can have a wide range of applications for orthopedic medicine. Their differentiation ability, easy manipulation in vitro, and relatively easy accessibility from various tissues enable them to become major building blocks for the design and development of therapeutic applications to all skeletal tissues concerned in orthopedics. It is expected that the use of MSCs will expand to other tissues and will acquire an important place in regenerative medicine.

References

1. Odorico JS, Kaufman DS, Thomson JA (2001) Multilineage differentiation from human embryonic stem cell lines. Stem Cells 19(3):193–204
2. Jiang Y, Jahagirdar BN, Reinhardt RL et al (2002) Pluripotency of mesenchymal stem cells derived from adult marrow. Nature 418(6893):41–49
3. Labat ML (2001) Stem cells and the promise of eternal youth: embryonic versus adult stem cells. Biomed Pharmacother 55(4):179–185
4. Martin JA, Buckwalter JA (2002) Aging, articular cartilage chondrocyte senescence and osteoarthritis. Biogerontology 3(5):257–264
5. Martin JA, Buckwalter JA (2002) Human chondrocyte senescence and osteoarthritis. Biorheology 39(1–2):145–152
6. Prockop DJ (1997) Marrow stromal cells as stem cells for nonhematopoietic tissues. Science 276(5309):71–74
7. Liu ZJ, Zhuge Y, Velazquez OC (2009) Trafficking and differentiation of mesenchymal stem cells. J Cell Biochem 106(6):984–991
8. Pittenger MF, Mackay AM, Beck SC et al (1999) Multilineage potential of adult human mesenchymal stem cells. Science 284(5411):143–147
9. Liechty KW, MacKenzie TC, Shaaban AF et al (2000) Human mesenchymal stem cells engraft and demonstrate site-specific differentiation after in utero transplantation in sheep. Nat Med 6(11):1282–1286
10. Jankowski RJ, Deasy BM, Huard J (2002) Muscle-derived stem cells. Gene Ther 9(10):642–647
11. Lin G, Garcia M, Ning H et al (2008) Defining stem and progenitor cells within adipose tissue. Stem Cells Dev 17(6):1053–1063
12. Gazit D, Turgeman G, Kelley P et al (1999) Engineered pluripotent mesenchymal cells integrate and differentiate in regenerating bone: a novel cell-mediated gene therapy. J Gene Med 1(2):121–133
13. Lieberman JR, Le LQ, Wu L et al (1998) Regional gene therapy with a BMP-2-producing murine stromal cell line induces heterotopic and orthotopic bone formation in rodents. J Orthop Res 16(3):330–339

14. Lou J, Xu F, Merkel K, Manske P (1999) Gene therapy: adenovirus-mediated human bone morphogenetic protein-2 gene transfer induces mesenchymal progenitor cell proliferation and differentiation in vitro and bone formation in vivo. J Orthop Res 17(1):43–50
15. Engstrand T, Daluiski A, Bahamonde ME, Melhus H, Lyons KM (2000) Transient production of bone morphogenetic protein 2 by allogeneic transplanted transduced cells induces bone formation. Hum Gene Ther 11(1):205–211
16. Lieberman JR, Daluiski A, Stevenson S et al (1999) The effect of regional gene therapy with bone morphogenetic protein-2-producing bone-marrow cells on the repair of segmental femoral defects in rats. J Bone Joint Surg Am 81(7):905–917
17. Hasharoni A, Zilberman Y, Turgeman G, Helm GA, Liebergall M, Gazit D (2005) Murine spinal fusion induced by engineered mesenchymal stem cells that conditionally express bone morphogenetic protein-2. J Neurosurg Spine 3(1):47–52
18. Wozney JM (2002) Overview of bone morphogenetic proteins. Spine 27((16 Suppl 1)):S2–S8
19. Ebara S, Nakayama K (2002) Mechanism for the action of bone morphogenetic proteins and regulation of their activity. Spine 27(16 (Suppl 1)):S10–S15
20. Yamaguchi A, Ishizuya T, Kintou N et al (1996) Effects of BMP-2, BMP-4, and BMP-6 on osteoblastic differentiation of bone marrow-derived stromal cell lines, ST2 and MC3T3-G2/PA6. Biochem Biophys Res Commun 220(2):366–371
21. Wang EA, Rosen V, D'Alessandro JS et al (1990) Recombinant human bone morphogenetic protein induces bone formation. Proc Natl Acad Sci USA 87(6):2220–2224
22. Volek-Smith H, Urist MR (1996) Recombinant human bone morphogenetic protein (rhBMP) induced heterotopic bone development in vivo and in vitro. Proc Soc Exp Biol Med 211(3):265–272
23. Hanada K, Dennis JE, Caplan AI (1997) Stimulatory effects of basic fibroblast growth factor and bone morphogenetic protein-2 on osteogenic differentiation of rat bone marrow-derived mesenchymal stem cells. J Bone Miner Res 12(10):1606–1614
24. Gori F, Thomas T, Hicok KC, Spelsberg TC, Riggs BL (1999) Differentiation of human marrow stromal precursor cells: bone morphogenetic protein-2 increases OSF2/CBFA1, enhances osteoblast commitment, and inhibits late adipocyte maturation. J Bone Miner Res 14(9):1522–1535
25. Fromigue O, Marie PJ, Lomri A (1998) Bone morphogenetic protein-2 and transforming growth factor-beta2 interact to modulate human bone marrow stromal cell proliferation and differentiation. J Cell Biochem 68(4):411–426
26. Chaudhari A, Ron E, Rethman MP (1997) Recombinant human bone morphogenetic protein-2 stimulates differentiation in primary cultures of fetal rat calvarial osteoblasts. Mol Cell Biochem 167(1–2):31–39
27. Wozney JM, Rosen V, Celeste AJ et al (1988) Novel regulators of bone formation: molecular clones and activities. Science 242(4885):1528–1534
28. Lecanda F, Avioli LV, Cheng SL (1997) Regulation of bone matrix protein expression and induction of differentiation of human osteoblasts and human bone marrow stromal cells by bone morphogenetic protein-2. J Cell Biochem 67(3):386–396
29. Steinhardt Y, Aslan H, Regev E et al (2008) Maxillofacial-derived stem cells regenerate critical mandibular bone defect. Tissue Eng Part A 14(11):1763–1773
30. Kirker-Head C, Karageorgiou V, Hofmann S et al (2007) BMP-silk composite matrices heal critically sized femoral defects. Bone 41(2):247–255
31. Wright V, Peng H, Usas A et al (2002) BMP4-expressing muscle-derived stem cells differentiate into osteogenic lineage and improve bone healing in immunocompetent mice. Mol Ther 6(2):169–178
32. Peng H, Wright V, Usas A et al (2002) Synergistic enhancement of bone formation and healing by stem cell-expressed VEGF and bone morphogenetic protein-4. J Clin Invest 110(6):751–759
33. Gysin R, Wergedal JE, Sheng MH et al (2002) Ex vivo gene therapy with stromal cells transduced with a retroviral vector containing the BMP4 gene completely heals critical size calvarial defect in rats. Gene Ther 9(15):991–999

34. Dumont RJ, Dayoub H, Li JZ et al (2002) Ex vivo bone morphogenetic protein-9 gene therapy using human mesenchymal stem cells induces spinal fusion in rodents. Neurosurgery 51(5):1239–1244, discussion 1244–1235

35. Chen Y, Cheung KM, Kung HF, Leong JC, Lu WW, Luk KD (2002) In vivo new bone formation by direct transfer of adenoviral-mediated bone morphogenetic protein-4 gene. Biochem Biophys Res Commun 298(1):121–127

36. Valdes M, Moore DC, Palumbo M et al (2007) rhBMP-6 stimulated osteoprogenitor cells enhance posterolateral spinal fusion in the New Zealand white rabbit. Spine J 7(3):318–325

37. Yoon ST, Boden SD (2002) Osteoinductive molecules in orthopaedics: basic science and preclinical studies. Clin Orthop Relat Res 395:33–43

38. Valentin-Opran A, Wozney J, Csimma C, Lilly L, Riedel GE (2002) Clinical evaluation of recombinant human bone morphogenetic protein-2. Clin Orthop Relat Res 395:110–120

39. Bishop GB, Einhorn TA (2007) Current and future clinical applications of bone morphogenetic proteins in orthopaedic trauma surgery. Int Orthop 31(6):721–727

40. Moutsatsos IK, Turgeman G, Zhou S et al (2001) Exogenously regulated stem cell-mediated gene therapy for bone regeneration. Mol Ther 3(4):449–461

41. Turgeman G, Pittman DD, Muller R et al (2001) Engineered human mesenchymal stem cells: a novel platform for skeletal cell mediated gene therapy. J Gene Med 3(3):240–251

42. Oreffo RO, Virdi AS, Triffitt JT (2001) Retroviral marking of human bone marrow fibroblasts: in vitro expansion and localization in calvarial sites after subcutaneous transplantation in vivo. J Cell Physiol 186(2):201–209

43. Bruder SP, Kurth AA, Shea M, Hayes WC, Jaiswal N, Kadiyala S (1998) Bone regeneration by implantation of purified, culture-expanded human mesenchymal stem cells. J Orthop Res 16(2):155–162

44. Mankani MH, Kuznetsov SA, Fowler B, Kingman A, Robey PG (2001) In vivo bone formation by human bone marrow stromal cells: effect of carrier particle size and shape. Biotechnol Bioeng 72(1):96–107

45. Laurencin CT, Attawia MA, Lu LQ et al (2001) Poly(lactide-co-glycolide)/hydroxyapatite delivery of BMP-2-producing cells: a regional gene therapy approach to bone regeneration. Biomaterials 22(11):1271–1277

46. Young BH, Peng H, Huard J (2002) Muscle-based gene therapy and tissue engineering to improve bone healing. Clin Orthop Relat Res 403 (Suppl):S243–S251

47. Skillington J, Choy L, Derynck R (2002) Bone morphogenetic protein and retinoic acid signaling cooperate to induce osteoblast differentiation of preadipocytes. J Cell Biol 159(1):135–146

48. Peterson B, Zhang J, Iglesias R et al (2005) Healing of critically sized femoral defects, using genetically modified mesenchymal stem cells from human adipose tissue. Tissue Eng 11(1–2):120–129

49. Musgrave DS, Pruchnic R, Bosch P, Ziran BH, Whalen J, Huard J (2002) Human skeletal muscle cells in ex vivo gene therapy to deliver bone morphogenetic protein-2. J Bone Joint Surg Br 84(1):120–127

50. Lee JY, Musgrave D, Pelinkovic D et al (2001) Effect of bone morphogenetic protein-2-expressing muscle-derived cells on healing of critical-sized bone defects in mice. J Bone Joint Surg Am 83-A(7):1032–1039

51. Dragoo JL, Choi JY, Lieberman JR et al (2003) Bone induction by BMP-2 transduced stem cells derived from human fat. J Orthop Res 21(4):622–629

52. De Ugarte DA, Morizono K, Elbarbary A et al (2003) Comparison of multi-lineage cells from human adipose tissue and bone marrow. Cells Tissues Organs 174(3):101–109

53. Usas A, Ho AM, Cooper GM, Olshanski A, Peng H, Huard J (2008) Bone regeneration mediated by BMP4-expressing muscle-derived stem cells is affected by delivery system. Tissue Eng Part A 15(2):285–293

54. Knippenberg M, Helder MN, Doulabi BZ, Bank RA, Wuisman PI, Klein-Nulend J (2009) Differential effects of bone morphogenetic protein-2 and transforming growth factor-beta1 on

gene expression of collagen-modifying enzymes in human adipose tissue-derived mesenchymal stem cells. Tissue Eng Part A 15(8):2213–2225

55. Hsu WK, Wang JC, Liu NQ et al (2008) Stem cells from human fat as cellular delivery vehicles in an athymic rat posterolateral spine fusion model. J Bone Joint Surg Am 90(5):1043–1052

56. Wobus AM, Boheler KR (1999) Embryonic Stem Cells as Developmental Model in vitro. Preface. Cells Tissues Organs 165(3–4):129–130

57. Phillips BW, Belmonte N, Vernochet C, Ailhaud G, Dani C (2001) Compactin enhances osteogenesis in murine embryonic stem cells. Biochem Biophys Res Commun 284(2):478–484

58. Karner E, Unger C, Sloan AJ, Ahrlund-Richter L, Sugars RV, Wendel M (2007) Bone matrix formation in osteogenic cultures derived from human embryonic stem cells in vitro. Stem Cells Dev 16(1):39–52

59. Robertson JA (2001) Human embryonic stem cell research: ethical and legal issues. Nat Rev Genet 2(1):74–78

60. Scott CT (2008) Stem cells: new frontiers of ethics, law, and policy. Neurosurg Focus 24(3–4):E24

61. Jiang Y, Vaessen B, Lenvik T, Blackstad M, Reyes M, Verfaillie CM (2002) Multipotent progenitor cells can be isolated from postnatal murine bone marrow, muscle, and brain. Exp Hematol 30(8):896–904

62. Kempen DH, Lu L, Heijink A et al (2009) Effect of local sequential VEGF and BMP-2 delivery on ectopic and orthotopic bone regeneration. Biomaterials 30(14):2816–2825

63. Gerber HP, Vu TH, Ryan AM, Kowalski J, Werb Z, Ferrara N (1999) VEGF couples hypertrophic cartilage remodeling, ossification and angiogenesis during endochondral bone formation. Nat Med 5(6):623–628

64. Yang X, Castilla LH, Xu X et al (1999) Angiogenesis defects and mesenchymal apoptosis in mice lacking SMAD5. Development 126(8):1571–1580

65. Yamashita H, Shimizu A, Kato M et al (1997) Growth/differentiation factor-5 induces angiogenesis in vivo. Exp Cell Res 235(1):218–226

66. David L, Feige JJ, Bailly S (2009) Emerging role of bone morphogenetic proteins in angiogenesis. Cytokine Growth Factor Rev 20(3):203–212

67. Peng H, Usas A, Olshanski A et al (2005) VEGF improves, whereas sFlt1 inhibits, BMP2-induced bone formation and bone healing through modulation of angiogenesis. J Bone Miner Res 20(11):2017–2027

68. Notelovitz M (1997) Estrogen therapy and osteoporosis: principles & practice. Am J Med Sci 313(1):2–12

69. Kassem M, Melton LJ, Riggs BL (1996) The type I/type II model for involutional osteoporosis. In: Marcus R, Feldman D, Kelsey J (eds) Osteoporosis. Academic, New York, pp 691–702

70. Turgeman G, Zilberman Y, Zhou S et al (2002) Systemically administered rhBMP-2 promotes MSC activity and reverses bone and cartilage loss in osteopenic mice. J Cell Biochem 86(3):461–474

71. Gazit D, Zilberman Y, Turgeman G, Zhou S, Kahn A (1999) Recombinant TGF-beta1 stimulates bone marrow osteoprogenitor cell activity and bone matrix synthesis in osteopenic, old male mice. J Cell Biochem 73(3):379–389

72. Gazit D, Zilberman Y, Ebner R, Kahn A (1998) Bone loss (osteopenia) in old male mice results from diminished activity and availability of TGF-beta. J Cell Biochem 70(4):478–488

73. Byers RJ, Hoyland JA, Braidman IP (2001) Osteoporosis in men: a cellular endocrine perspective of an increasingly common clinical problem. J Endocrinol 168(3):353–362

74. Bellantuono I, Aldahmash A, Kassem M (2009) Aging of marrow stromal (skeletal) stem cells and their contribution to age-related bone loss. Biochim Biophys Acta 1792(4):364–370

75. Zhou S, Zilberman Y, Wassermann K, Bain SD, Sadovsky Y, Gazit D (2001) Estrogen modulates estrogen receptor alpha and beta expression, osteogenic activity, and apoptosis in mesenchymal stem cells (MSCs) of osteoporotic mice. J Cell Biochem Suppl 36 (Suppl):144–155

76. Goater JJ, O'Keefe RJ, Rosier RN, Puzas JE, Schwarz EM (2002) Efficacy of ex vivo OPG gene therapy in preventing wear debris induced osteolysis. J Orthop Res 20(2):169–173

77. Yudoh K, Matsuno H, Nakazawa F, Katayama R, Kimura T (2001) Reconstituting telomerase activity using the telomerase catalytic subunit prevents the telomere shorting and replicative senescence in human osteoblasts. J Bone Miner Res 16(8):1453–1464

78. Murray J (1999) Primer on the metabolic bone diseases and disorders of mineral metabolism. Lippincott Williams & Wilkins, Philadelphia

79. Abboud SL, Woodruff K, Liu C, Shen V, Ghosh-Choudhury N (2002) Rescue of the osteopetrotic defect in op/op mice by osteoblast-specific targeting of soluble colony-stimulating factor-1. Endocrinology 143(5):1942–1949

80. Niyibizi C, Smith P, Mi Z, Phillips CL, Robbins P (2001) Transfer of proalpha2(I) cDNA into cells of a murine model of human Osteogenesis Imperfecta restores synthesis of type I collagen comprised of alpha1(I) and alpha2(I) heterotrimers in vitro and in vivo. J Cell Biochem 83(1):84–91

81. Kuhlcke K, Fehse B, Schilz A et al (2002) Highly efficient retroviral gene transfer based on centrifugation-mediated vector preloading of tissue culture vessels. Mol Ther 5(4):473–478

82. Sugiyama O, An DS, Kung SP et al (2005) Lentivirus-mediated gene transfer induces long-term transgene expression of BMP-2 in vitro and new bone formation in vivo. Mol Ther 11(3):390–398

83. Miyazaki M, Sugiyama O, Zou J et al (2008) Comparison of lentiviral and adenoviral gene therapy for spinal fusion in rats. Spine (Phila Pa 1976) 33(13):1410–1417

84. Liu P, Kalajzic I, Stover ML, Rowe DW, Lichtler AC (2001) Human bone marrow stromal cells are efficiently transduced by vesicular stomatitis virus-pseudotyped retrovectors without affecting subsequent osteoblastic differentiation. Bone 29(4):331–335

85. Kalajzic I, Stover ML, Liu P, Kalajzic Z, Rowe DW, Lichtler AC (2001) Use of VSV-G pseudotyped retroviral vectors to target murine osteoprogenitor cells. Virology 284(1):37–45

86. Ricks DM, Kutner R, Zhang XY, Welsh DA, Reiser J (2008) Optimized lentiviral transduction of mouse bone marrow-derived mesenchymal stem cells. Stem Cells Dev 17(3):441–450

87. Peng H, Chen ST, Wergedal JE et al (2001) Development of an MFG-based retroviral vector system for secretion of high levels of functionally active human BMP4. Mol Ther 4(2):95–104

88. Stover ML, Wang CK, McKinstry MB et al (2001) Bone-directed expression of Col1a1 promoter-driven self-inactivating retroviral vector in bone marrow cells and transgenic mice. Mol Ther 3(4):543–550

89. Kuznetsov SA, Mankani MH, Gronthos S, Satomura K, Bianco P, Robey PG (2001) Circulating skeletal stem cells. J Cell Biol 153(5):1133–1140

90. Viggeswarapu M, Boden SD, Liu Y et al (2001) Adenoviral delivery of LIM mineralization protein-1 induces new-bone formation in vitro and in vivo. J Bone Joint Surg Am 83-A(3):364–376

91. Varady P, Li JZ, Cunningham M et al (2001) Morphologic analysis of BMP-9 gene therapy-induced osteogenesis. Hum Gene Ther 12(6):697–710

92. Griffith CK, Miller C, Sainson RC et al (2005) Diffusion limits of an in vitro thick prevascularized tissue. Tissue Eng 11(1–2):257–266

93. Bouchentouf M, Benabdallah BF, Bigey P, Yau TM, Scherman D, Tremblay JP (2008) Vascular endothelial growth factor reduced hypoxia-induced death of human myoblasts and improved their engraftment in mouse muscles. Gene Ther 15(6):404–414

94. Potier E, Ferreira E, Andriamanalijaona R et al (2007) Hypoxia affects mesenchymal stromal cell osteogenic differentiation and angiogenic factor expression. Bone 40(4):1078–1087

95. Fang TD, Salim A, Xia W et al (2005) Angiogenesis is required for successful bone induction during distraction osteogenesis. J Bone Miner Res 20(7):1114–1124

96. Riess JG (2006) Perfluorocarbon-based oxygen delivery. Artif Cells Blood Substit Immobil Biotechnol 34(6):567–580

97. Lowe KC, Davey MR, Power JB (1998) Perfluorochemicals: their applications and benefits to cell culture. Trends Biotechnol 16(6):272–277

98. Kimelman-Bleich N, Pelled G, Sheyn D et al (2009) The use of a synthetic oxygen carrier-enriched hydrogel to enhance mesenchymal stem cell-based bone formation in vivo. Biomaterials 30(27):4639–4648

Chapter 8
Scaffolds in Skeletal Repair

Erella Livne and Samer Srouji

The need for tissue repair is one of the major concerns of reconstructive surgery and in aging and disease. Fracture healing is regulated by osteogenic cells and growth factors. The ability to enhance healing of bone defects and fractures can contribute to prevent the complications of long-term immobilization that are especially fatal in old age. Three-dimensional scaffold provides the necessary support for cells to proliferate and maintain their differentiated function and its architecture defines the shape of the newly formed bone. At the same time the scaffold is biodegraded providing space for the newly formed tissue. Skeletal tissue such as bone is organized into three-dimensional structure (3D) in the body. The 3D scaffold can be used as a temporary device containing the osteogenic cells. This could provide the initial conditions for bone repair. Biodegradable scaffold contains committed osteogenic stem cells and growth factors which serve as a graft substitute for bone and cartilage repair. Bone marrow stem cells are selected as the osteogenic subpopulations cultured in medium supplemented with osteogenic supplements. The selected osteogenic subpopulation is identified using osteogenic markers (Alizarin red, von Kossa staining, osteocalcin, osteonectin, osteopontin immunolocalization, and mineral-hydroxyapatite (HA) deposition). Committed osteoprogenitor cells are cultured on scaffold and transplanted with growth factors in tibia segmental bone defect. The healing of the defect is examined by morphology, radiology, 3D CT, and EDS for mineral deposition. Results indicated that our 3D hydrogel scaffold supports proliferation and differentiation of bone marrow stem cells. This provides an approach for the use of bone marrow stem cells-based transplants of bone cells that will enhance bone repair, eliminate the need for additional surgical procedure, reduce unnecessary pain and complications to the patient, and shorten the hospitalization time. The biodegradable scaffold can serve as biocompatible matrix for bone marrow stem

E. Livne (✉) • S. Srouji
Technion-Israel Institute of Technology, Haifa, Israel
e-mail: livne@tx.technion.ac.il; mdsamer@technion.ac.il

J.J. Sela and I.A. Bab (eds.), *Principles of Bone Regeneration*,
DOI 10.1007/978-1-4614-2059-0_8, © Springer Science+Business Media, LLC 2012

cells-derived osteoprogenitor cells and growth factors, and that it also provides space for bone regeneration. The biodegradable scaffold containing committed stem cells and growth factors is thus a promising surgical tool for enhancement of bone and cartilage defect reconstruction for tissue engineering in aging and disease. Fracture healing is regulated by osteogenic cells and growth factors. The ability to enhance healing of bone defects and fractures can contribute to prevent the complications of long-term immobilization that are especially fatal in old age [1]. Skeletal tissue such as bone is organized into three-dimensional (3D) structure in the body. The search for artificial bone graft can contribute to the enhancement of bone repair. Scaffolds are 3D structures used as bone graft substitute for bone repair. The (3D) structure scaffold provides the necessary support for cells to proliferate and maintain their differentiated function, and its architecture defines the shape of the newly formed bone. At the same time the scaffold is biodegraded providing space for the newly formed tissue [2–4]. Bone is the second most frequently transplanted tissue in humans. Surgical uses of bone grafting materials include surgical intervention of osseous nonunion, restoration of the structural integrity of bone after trauma, and filling defects following bone tumor removal. Autogenous cancellous bone is considered the ideal graft material for several reasons: it is biocompatible and nonimmunogenic, it will not transmit a disease to a recipient, and it has osteogenic potential due to the presence of viable osteoprogenitor cells [5, 6]. Since cancellous bone is taken from the iliac crest, rib, fibula, or tibia, it is sometimes not available in a sufficient amount. In addition, harvesting the bone imposes potential complications of pain, blood loss, infection, and donor site instability. Another frequently used bone graft material is allogenous bone. Allograft bone is available in an unlimited supply but, unfortunately, does not have the osteogenic potential of the autogenous bone and often elicits immunological response when implanted. This leads to continued search for effective artificial substitutes for bone grafts [7, 8]. The stromal compartment bone is composed of a network of interconnected stromal cells that include mesenchymal stem cells (MSCs), distinct from the hematopoietic stem cells (HSCs). The MSCs are capable of differentiating along the osteogenic, chondrogenic, fibroblastic, and adipogenic lineages. MSCs-derived osteoprogenitor cells can be used in modern technology for tissue engineering and cell therapy. They can be used in metabolic bone diseases and orthopedic approaches when bone repair is needed. By accomplishing the task of identifying a specific osteoprogenitors, the selection of osteoprogenitor cells from the bone marrow will be available [9, 10]. The development of an osteoinductive slow-release devices containing committed bone forming cells and growth factors will minimize the need for autologous bone grafts used today for filling bone voids or gaps, and will thereby reduce the inherent risks and complications associated with the additional surgery of bone harvesting [11, 12]. Reinforcing the developed osteogenic bone graft substitute will improve the mechanical properties of the device thereby extending its potential applications to highly loaded locations in the human body. Introduction of such bone substitute into clinical practice will restore the mobility and improve the quality of life of both young and aging patients who lost bone during trauma or surgical resection [13]. Biodegradable scaffold can serve as a biocompatible matrix for bone marrow stem

Fig. 8.1 Strategy for bone
repair using cell-scaffold
constructs

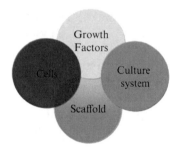

cells-derived osteoprogenitor cells and growth factors, and that it also provides space for bone regeneration (Fig. 8.1). The biodegradable scaffold containing committed stem cells and growth factors is thus a promising surgical tool for enhancement of bone and cartilage defect reconstruction for tissue engineering in aging and disease [14].

8.1   Bone Defect Repair and Growth Factors

The need for bone repair is one of the major concerns in bone defects, fracture healing, and reconstructive surgery [15, 16]. Bone consists of cells and extracellular matrix; the latter is comprised of 35% organic and 65% inorganic components [17]. The inorganic components are mainly calcium and phosphate as HA. The organic components of bone matrix are traditionally divided into collagen and non-collagenous proteins. Type I collagen constitutes more than 90% of the organic material in bone matrix and is the major structural protein of bone. The remaining 10%, the non-collagenous proteins, have different regulatory functions for mineralization, mediation of cell matrix-to-matrix binding, and various interactions with structural proteins such as collagen. Bone silaoprotein (BSP) is involved in calcium binding [18]. Bone growth factors consist of less than 1% of the non-collagenous proteins. The main cell types in bone include the osteoblast, osteocyte, and osteoclast. The process of bone remodeling is regulated by osteoblast–osteoclast direct signaling [19–21]. The bone growth factors exhibit their effect in local cellular environments, thereby stimulating neighboring bone cells to proliferate and increase matrix protein synthesis (paracrine effect). Likewise, the osteoblast which produces the growth factors can stimulate themselves to additional metabolic activity (autocrine effect). The total number of growth factors which are able to affect proliferation, differentiation, and secretive functions of bone-related cells is unknown [17] (Fig. 8.1). In 1965, in an experiment to recalcify cortical bone, Marshall Urist [22] made the key discovery that led to the hunt for factors responsible for bone formation. Urist's discovery led to a series of investigation to determine the putative agents in demineralized bone (DMB) that provoke autoinduction. The osteoinduction activity in bone matrix was found to be the result of non-collagenous and water soluble substance coined bone morphogenetic proteins (BMPs) [23]. BMPs are members of the transforming growth factor-β (TGF-β) superfamily and regulate differentiation of various cells implicated in cartilage and bone formation during skeletal development and fracture repair [24, 25]. The role of BMPs in induction of osteoblast differentiation has been established using various preosteoblastic cell lines, such as primary cultures of calvarial osteoblasts and human and mouse bone marrow cultures. Using these models, induction of osteoblast differentiation has been described for BMP-2, -4, -5, -6, and -7 [26–29]. BMPs exert their effect by binding to a heterodimeric complex, consisting of two BMP type I receptors and two BMP type II receptors, which possesses serine/threonine kinase activity.. To date, however, it is still not clear how BMPs being potentially a big promise, failed to play a larger role in the clinical arena. Other local growth factors have proven to be important by affecting the type and the rate of fracture repair. An age-related diminished capacity of fracture repair process has been observed with the advancement of aging and an overall decrease in osteoblast function was observed with aging [30]. Nielsen et al. [31] reported on increase in bone strength of tibial fracture following local injection of TGF-β (40 ng, every second day for up to 40 days) and an ultimate load dose-dependent increase in cross-sectional area of callus and bone at the fracture line. However, in a study on distraction TGF-β had no detectable effect on bone mineral density or bone volume in the distraction gap, but increased fibrous tissue in the callus region. Another study on mid-tibial osteotomy in rabbits treated with TGF-β1 (10 ng/day for 6 weeks) resulted in increased maximal bending strength and callus formation [32]. IGF-1 is known to play a role in fracture healing; it promotes cell proliferation and matrix synthesis by chondrocytes and osteoblasts. The levels of circulating IGF-1 and bone mineral density decrease with the increase in age. Also the secretion of GH decreases with aging [33]. It has been shown that administration of IGF-1 increased bone turnover in patients with low bone mineral density. FGF-2 was also shown to stimulate callus formation which provided mechanical stability to the fracture, accelerated healing, and restored competence [34, 35]. Also increased bone mineral content and osteoblast number were observed in fracture healing in dogs treated with FGF-2 [36] and in rabbit skull defect [37] (Fig. 8.2).

Fracture healing is a process of reconstruction of the tissue. The matrix in the fracture and in the defect sites plays an effective role in the earlier restoration of the mechanical strength. A process of remodeling occurs and the molecular mediators released by the aggregating platelets and other thrombotic factors, as well as active mediators, are released by the tissue breakdown. All these structures produce many factors such as chemo-attractants, angiogenic and growth factors. The monocytes and macrophages that exist in the hematoma, or infiltrate to the infected site also produce growth factors involved in bone repair. The platelets contain several growth factors such as platelets-derived growth factor (PDGF), epidermal growth factor (EGF), TGF-β, and many others. Different blood cells (granulocytes, macrophages, and erythrocytes) migrate in waves to the fracture site [38, 39] and to supply the various factors that are in involved in bone repair process. No knowledge of the constituents of the fracture exudates is available, but it is known that the fracture

Fig. 8.2 Involvement of various growth factors in proliferation and differentiation of skeletal progenitor cells along the osteoblastic lineage

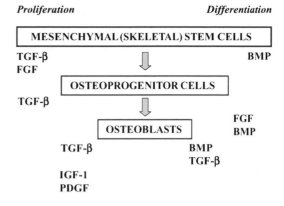

Proliferation   *Differentiation*

| MESENCHYMAL (SKELETAL) STEM CELLS |

TGF-β   BMP
FGF   ⇩

| OSTEOPROGENITOR CELLS |

TGF-β   ⇩

                                                              FGF
                        | OSTEOBLASTS | BMP

        TGF-β   BMP
                                           TGF-β

        IGF-1
        PDGF

callus contains a high amount of hyaluronate in the beginning which decreases after 7–8 days. Hyaluronate promotes migration and proliferation of mesenchymal cells. It is likely that growth factors regulate both resorption and formation of bone in remodeling process. TGF-β seems to be of special importance in fracture healing and induces the typical granulation tissue [40]. In the present study, TGF-β and the combination of TGF-β + IGF-1 were shown to induce bone defect healing. It is hypothesized that growth factors and selected bone forming cells that will be incorporated in osteoinductive osteoconductive scaffold will enhance bone formation. The scaffold with appropriate biodegradability will function not only as a release matrix for the growth factors and cells, but also as a space provided for bone osseointegration affecting the firmness of the external fixation implants. The hydrogel containing growth factors and bone forming cells is thus a promising surgical tool for bone defects and for orthopedic implants osseointegration. TGF-β may stimulate bone repair by causing proliferation of osteoblasts or by stimulating mineralization as represented by expression of alkaline phosphatase [41, 42]. TGF-β influences osteoblast production of several bone proteins like osteonectin, a bone-specific 32 K protein linking mineral to collagen fibers, osteopontin, a matrix protein enhancing cell attachment, fibronectin, collagens, and proteoglycans. Two other ways in which TGF-β may enhance the formation of ECM are by stimulating the production of protease inhibitors such as plasminogen activator inhibitor (PAI), and tissue inhibitor of metalloproteases (TIMP), or by inhibiting the production of proteases such as plasminogen activator and metalloproteases. On the other hand, MMPs are needed for resorption of the initial callus and for remodeling of cancellous bone to compact bone. The process of bone resorption could serve also for the release of matrix-stored growth factors by bone resorption. Thus, osteoblasts deposit growth factors in bone and later when these growth factors are released from bone via bone resorption, the growth factors stimulate osteoblast precursors to proliferate [43, 44]. TGF-β plays also a role in the formation of new bone and bone repair by stimulation of collagen and matrix protein synthesis by bone cells and chondrocytes. It is concluded that TGF-β and TGF-β + IGF-1 were shown to induce an increase in the rate of bone defect repair process and restore the biomechanical quality of the newly formed tissue. Finding a treatment that can induce an increase in bone mass is important to enhance osteoinduction in bone defects loss and reconstructive surgery and aging [45, 46]. Bone defect healing depends on the mechanical stability and on the actual size of an osteotomy or bone defect [47]. The relationship between biomechanical properties and bone formation during the healing of the defect revealed that after 2 weeks the biomechanical tests did not reveal yet any significant changes between the groups and the control. At the same time, the morphology did not reveal new bone formation. Moreover, the biomechanical changes of the various treatments and of the control were significantly different from the intact femur. After 4 weeks, the biomechanical properties of the bones treated with TGF-β+IGF-1 were different from the other treatments and were closer to the value of the intact femur, and at the same time morphology revealed that cancellous bone was present in the defect site [45, 48, 49]. Radiology revealed that after 2 weeks some opacity was seen in the TGF-β+IGF-1 group. It represents the very beginning of response to the growth factor, but not enough to be seen in the mechanical tests.

8.2 Bone Marrow Stem Cells

The human skeleton accumulates bone up to approximately age 30, after which bone is gradually lost. Bone remodeling and bone loss as a function of age are under the influence of both endogenous hormonal changes and external mechanical loads resulting from physical activity. These impart their effects through regulation of the relative activities of bone cells in particular osteoblasts and osteoclasts, which control bone deposition and resorption, respectively [50, 51]. The need for bone repair is one of the major concerns of reconstructive surgery and fractures [52, 53]. Fracture healing is regulated by osteogenic cells and systemic growth factors. To aid the healing process, it is often necessary to introduce the selective subpopulation of bone forming osteoprogenitor cells in the healing bone tissue. Bone grafts are currently being used for repair of large defects and fractures, and bone grafting should improve recovery, shorten hospitalization time, and decrease complication frequency [54, 55]. Bone marrow MSCs are multipotent cells capable of forming bone, cartilage, and other connective tissues. These cells may also provide a potential therapy for bone repair [56, 57]. It has been well documented that MSCs include actively proliferating osteoprogenitor cells [58–61]. In vitro, these cells express the osteogenic phenotype only when treated with differentiation factors such as glucocorticoids [62–64]. Maniatopoulos et al. described a culture system in which MSCs obtained from bone marrow of fetal or neonatal skeleton have the capacity to produce mineralized-like nodules in vitro when the culture medium is supplemented with dexamethasone, ascorbic acid, and β-glycerophosphate [63]. The ECM secreted by MSC in this culture system was shown to consist predominantly of type I collagen, to include osteonectin and osteocalcin, to contain bone hydroxyapatite as its mineral phase, and to express BMPs [63]. These properties are characteristic of bone ECM produced in vivo. The differentiation of osteoblast, to bone-like tissue, has been muddled as three-step process, consisting of proliferation phase, a matrix maturation phase, and mineralization phase [65]. Adult stem cells, like all stem cells, share at least two characteristics. First, they can make identical copies of themselves for long periods of time; this ability to proliferate is referred to as long-term self-renewal. Second, they can give rise to mature cell types that have characteristic morphologies and specialized functions. Typically, stem cells generate an intermediate cell type or types before they achieve their fully differentiated state. The intermediate cell is called a precursor or progenitor cell. Progenitor or precursor cells in fetal or adult tissues are partly differentiated cells that divide and give rise to differentiated cells. Such cells are usually regarded as "committed" to differentiating along a particular cellular development pathway, although this characteristic may not be as definitive as once though [14]. Adult stem cells are rare. Their primary functions are to maintain the steady-state functioning of a cell and, with limitations, to replace cells that die because of injury or disease [66]. For example, only an estimated 1 in 10,000 to 15,000 cells in the bone marrow is a HSC (blood forming) [67]. And 1 in 1:100,000 is estimated as osteoprogenitor stem cell. Furthermore, adult stem cells are dispersed in tissues throughout the mature animal and behave very differently, depending on their local environment [68]. Bone marrow stromal cells represent a mixed cell population that generates bone, cartilage, fat, fibrous connective tissue, and the reticular network that supports blood cell formation [2, 69, 70]. The bone marrow appears to contain three stem cell populations—HSCs, stromal cells, and (possibly) endothelial progenitor cells. To date, it has not been possible to isolate a population of pure stromal cells from bone marrow. Panels of markers used to identify the cells include receptors for certain cytokines (interleukin-1, 3, 4, 6, and 7), receptors for proteins in the extracellular matrix (ICAM-1 and 2, VCAM-1, the α-1, 2, and 3 integrins, and the β-1, 2, 3, and 4 integrins), etc. Despite the use of these markers and another stromal cell marker called Stro-1, the origin and specific identity of stromal cells have remained elusive. Like HSCs, stromal cells arise from embryonic mesoderm during development, although no specific precursor or stem cell for stromal cells has been isolated and identified [71].

8.3   Scaffolds and Biomaterials

There are many approaches to bone tissue engineering, but all involve one or more of the following key components: cultured stem cell, growth factors, and three-dimensional (3D) matrices. One approach involves seeding highly porous biodegradable matrices (or scaffolds), with cells and signaling molecules (e.g., protein growth factors), then culturing and implanting the scaffolds into the defect to induce and direct the growth of new bone [72, 73]. The goal for the cells is to attach to the scaffold, multiply, differentiate (i.e., transform from a nonspecific or primitive state

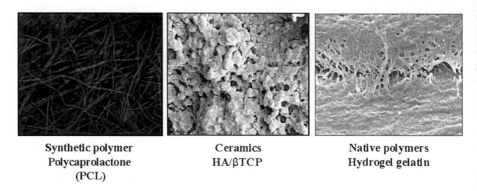

Synthetic polymer	Ceramics	Native polymers
Polycaprolactone	HA/βTCP	Hydrogel gelatin
(PCL)		

Fig. 8.3 Types of scaffolds for bone

into cells exhibiting the bone-specific functions), and organize into normal, healthy bone as the scaffold degrades. Scaffold materials for making matrices for bone tissue engineering include several classes of biomaterials: synthetic polymers, ceramics, native polymers, and composites (Fig. 8.3).

8.3.1 Synthetic Polymers

Both organic and inorganic are used in a wide variety of biomedical applications. The polymers can be biodegradable or nondegradable. Examples of biodegradable polymers include polylactic acid (PLA), polyglycolic acid (PLGA), and copolymers thereof. These polymers are broken down in the body hydrolytically to produce lactic acid and glycolic acid, respectively. Other biodegradable polymers currently being studied for tissue engineering applications include polycaprolactone (PCL), polyanhydrides, and polyphosphazenes [74–78].

8.3.2 Ceramics

These are widely used in dental applications and are being examined for bone tissue engineering applications. Two common ceramics used in dentistry and hip prostheses are alumina and HA. Alumina (Al_2O_3) has excellent corrosion resistance, good biocompatibility, high strength, and high wear resistance, and has been used for over 20 years in orthopedic surgery [79]. HA is a calcium phosphate-based ceramic and has also been used for over 20 years in medicine and dentistry [80]. HA is a major component of the inorganic compartment of bone. HA prepared commercially is biocompatible with biodegradability either absent or protracted [81, 82]. The degradation of HA can be controlled by varying the chemical structure. Tricalcium phosphate degrades much more quickly than HA [13] and has been used for long bone defects repair in rabbits [83, 84]. Bioactive glasses have been shown to bind to soft tissue and bone. These bioactive glasses contain different ratios of $Na_2O–CaO–P_2O_5–SiO_2$ [85]. There are currently two commercially available glasses advertised for applications in bone sites.

8.3.3   Native Polymers

These are extracellular matrix proteins commonly exploited as bone graft materials. Collagens, which comprise a majority of proteins in connective tissue such as skin, bone, cartilage, and tendons, are popular candidates for such circumstances, and various collagen-based products are currently under development [86–88]. The organic phase of bone is principally type I collagen. When bone is demineralized with hydrochloric acid, the method used by most commercial venders, the bone derivative is largely type I collagen and a minimal percent mixture of ECM components, cell debris, and soluble signaling molecules that are resistant to acidic demineralization [89–91]. The format for the DBM can be either a range of particulate matter, blocks, or strips.

8.3.4   Composites

The composites of ceramics and polymers are also widely studied. Composites can result in substitutes with properties between each of the respective materials [92]. For example, bovine collagen has been manufactured with HA. Collagraft is HA and bovine type I dermal collagen (95%) and type III collagen (5%). Collagraft is used for orthopedic, non-load bearing sites [93]. Bone repair is thought to be one of the first major applications of tissue engineering. At present, efforts are being made to encourage the growth of new bone, using novel matrices, growth factors, gene therapy, and stem cells [8]. Today bone grafts from elsewhere in the body to repair major damage from accidents or disease are being used, but the quality and quantity of bone is not sufficient and repair is not always achieved. Molecular scaffolds made of collagen and HA are used for small divots but are not useful for larger defects [94]. Biocompatible polymers containing growth factors were also studied, gene-cell therapy are being tested; however, cells carrying therapeutic genes are short lived [24, 94].

8.4   Bioreactors

Static cultures do not mimic the dynamics of the in vivo environment found in bone, namely the mechanical stimulation caused by hydrostatic pressure and shear stress. These factors do not affect the behavior of osteocyte at several levels [95].

Furthermore, it has been also demonstrated that mechanical stress could also upregulate Cbaf-1/runx2 expression [96].

The cultivation of cell monolayer in culture dishes to multiply the initial cell number has various disadvantages. The supply of oxygen becomes critical when the diffusion distance comes wider than 100–200 μm, and the diffusion can be improved by stirring the culture medium. The design and development of bioreactors are for sure solutions to overcome the above-referred problems [97]. Various types of bioreactors have been tested for their utility in bone tissue engineering. Two systems have been preferentially used, spinner flasks and rotating wall vessel reactor. The spinner flasks provide better migration of cells and supply of nutrients [5]. The approach of cell cultures scaffold in bioreactor will provide the optimal conditions for 3D structure scaffold/cell as bone.

8.5   Scaffold and Growth Factors for Segmental Bone Repair

Bone regeneration induced by TGF-β and IGF-1-containing hydrogel scaffold was investigated using a rat tibia defect model. An external fixation device was used before induction of the bone defect, thus enabling a controlled segmental bone defect to be created in the already fixed tibia. Soft X-rays of the defects in TGF-β-treated animals, taken after 2 weeks from start of treatment, revealed some radiopacity, indicative of newly formed mineralized bone. It has been demonstrated previously that TGF-β is ionically complexed with the hydrogel scaffold and was released from it [11, 87]. A similar effect was reported for bFGF released from hydrogel [98]. Other studies have shown that growth factors released from scaffolds induced similar responses, but only after 8 weeks [76]. Enhanced healing of bone defects is a challenge to surgery and requires a combination of the osteoinductive effect of growth factors and the conductivity of scaffolds [99]. Enhanced bone formation and bone healing could lead to improved results in surgical procedures [100, 101]. In our hydrogel system, TGF-β and IGF-1 were released from hydrogel as a result of hydrogel biodegradation. When hydrogel degrades too quickly, it neither retains its growth factors allowing in growth of soft tissue in the defect, nor does it induces bone regeneration, while hydrogel that degrades too slowly could impede the formation of new bone [88].

8.6   Scaffold Biodegradation

It has been reported that metalloproteinases (MMPs) are present in bone tissue [102]. It is possible that proteases such as MMPs capable of degrading the hydrogel scaffold are involved in biodegradation of the hydrogel and bone remodeling [103]. TGF-β has been reported to enhance fixation and ingrowth of ceramic [20] and HA [21] coated implants. However, further research is needed to establish the optimal conditions for bone defect healing in long bones.

It is concluded that scaffold containing growth factors with appropriate biode-gradability could function not only as a release matrix for growth factors but also as a site for bone osseointegration that affects the firmness of the external fixation implants. Therefore, scaffold containing growth factors appears to be a promising surgical tool for the treatment for orthopedic bone repair.

8.7   Bone Tissue Engineering

Bone repair is a process of reconstruction of the bone tissue in the area of injury. This process is mediated by bone forming osteoprogenitor cells, growth factors, and three-dimensional cell matrixes at the site of injury [104, 105]. The decrease in skeletal bone formation and rate of fracture repair observed with aging in bone defects and in osteoporosis has been suggested to be due to a decrease in the growth factors and reduced numbers of the osteogenic progenitors [50]. The need for bone repair is one of the major concerns in bone defects, fracture healing, and recon-structive surgery. The ability of selected bone forming cells or TGF-β1 and IGF-1 incorporated into gelatin hydrogel to induce bone regeneration were evaluated in a previous study [46]. The use of PLA–PLGA copolymer-gelatin sponge containing rhBMP-2 induced effective bone regeneration in a rat mandible defect model [78]. TGF-β and IGF-1 incorporated into hydrogel scaffold were released from the scaf-fold as a result of biodegradation. When the scaffold degrades too quickly, it does not retain its growth factors, thus allowing ingrowths of soft tissue at the defect site, and does not induce bone regeneration. Scaffold that degrades too slowly could impede the formation of new bone [98]. The scaffold has to be degraded in vivo allowing the slow release of its incorporated growth factors. It could thus serve as a slow-release device. At present, efforts are being made to encourage the growth of new bone using novel matrices, growth factors, and stem cells [8]. Growth factors are important mediators of bone regeneration, but in vivo growth factors are short lived. In order to increase the availability of growth factors at the site of bone healing, the use of growth factors together with scaffolds has been introduced. Various carriers such as guanidine-extracted DBM matrix, polymeric or ceramic implants, bone grafts, or human recombinant osteogenic protein-1 con-taining growth factors were tested and shown to result in induced bone repair in various systems [7, 106–108]. IGF-1 incorporated into type I collagen gel enhanced nasal defects healing, and TGF-β incorporated into acid gelatin hydrogel enhanced healing of rabbit skull defects [109–111] as well as in others [112–114]. In order to further increase the osteogenic potential of scaffold-based implants, a cell therapy approach is used to incorporate osteoprogenitor cell derived from bone marrow stem cells (MSCs) in the scaffold to enhance bone repair. Cell-scaffold constructs are used for testing the functionality of vivo bone repair by selected osteogenic subpopulation of bone marrow stem cells (MSCs). The results are validated using specific osteogenic markers [115, 116]. Culture of sufficient numbers of such osteo-genic cells and growth factors could conceivably be used with scaffold for bone

Electrospun 3D scaffold   3D hydrogel gelatin scaffold

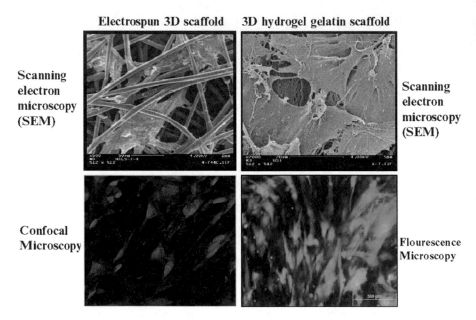

Fig. 8.4 Cell-scaffold constructs for bone repair

tissue engineering to repair bone in aging and in bone transplantation (Fig. 8.4). The methods used for in vitro selection of the osteogenic subpopulation from MSC cultures and the methods used to incorporate them in scaffold are crucial for the successful transplants for the future use in tissue engineering bone repair [5, 57, 90, 117–119]. The scaffold should be biocompatible for selected osteogenic cells and to provide support for proliferation and differentiation demonstrated by osteogenic markers. This approach can contribute to future development of an in vitro designed implant for in vivo bone repair. Scaffold should be biocompatible, osteoconductive, biodegradable, and osteinductive but not immunoreactive. Three-dimensional scaffolds should provide the necessary support for cells to proliferate and maintain their capacity to differentiate. The transition from the 2D culture system to the 3D scaffold provides a system that imitates the natural 3D structure of the body tissues and specifically the structure of bone. Three-dimensional scaffolds containing bone marrow-derived osteoprogenitors can be used within transplants in order to enhance bone repair. The complex construct is intended to mimic the native in vivo microenvironment, and this necessitates construction of bioactive scaffolds which are also capable of supporting vascularization as well as cell proliferation and osteogenic differentiation. Preclinical animal tests are a crucial step before conduction of the actual clinical trials. The preclinical tests are aimed for validation of the functionality of the transplanted cells, for safety tests, and for assessment of nonimmune reactivity of either the cells or the scaffold in the designed transplanted cell-scaffold constructs.

8.8   In Vivo Preclinical Tests

Animal testing constitutes a step midway between in vitro studies and human clinical applications. In vivo preclinical testing is crucial for the proof-of-functionality of the designed cell-scaffold constructs. Small animals used in preclinical studies are mice, rats, and rabbits. Mice are the most common animal models for molecular testing because their genome has been completely sequenced, and moreover immune-deficient mice strains (Nude, SCID beige) are used for testing human cells transplants in preclinical testing [4]. There are a number of different types of bone diseases and injuries. Known bone conditions include bone defects either cranial defect or long bone segmental defect as well as osteopenia (osteoporosis), osteonecrosis, bone fractures, and osteotomies (Fig. 8.5).

The most common tests are aimed for the repair of large voids, osteotomies, and critical size defects (CSDs) of bone. CSD was first described by Schmitz and Hollinger [52] as: "the smallest intraosseous wound that does not heal by bone formation during the lifetime of the animal," and later as: "defect which has less than 10% of bony regeneration occurring within the lifetime of the animal" [120]. The biofunctionality tests do not need to be evaluated in a complex biological and biomechanical environment reproducing clinical-like situations. Simple tests such as animal implantation in ectopic/heterotopic (subcutaneous, intramuscular), orthotopic (calvaria) sites allow in vivo evaluation of biocompatibility, osseointegration, osteoconductive, and osteogenic potential. On the contrary, preclinical evaluations rely on animal models simulating the clinical situation in which the bone replacement material will be used. The available models include long bone defect models, the radial, ulnar, femoral, and tibial bone defects, and post-transplants evaluations radiology, histology, μCT, and imunohistochemistry are performed for assessment of the results (Fig. 8.6)

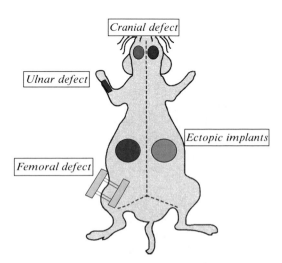

Fig. 8.5 Animal models for bone repair

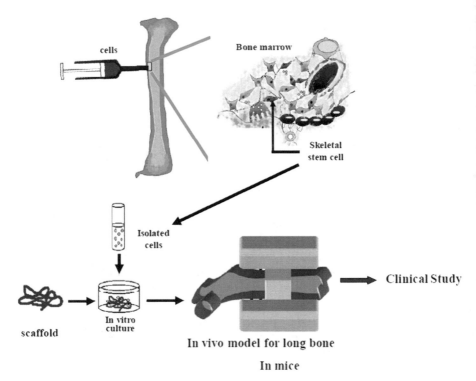

cells

Bone marrow

Skeletal
stem cell

Isolated
cells

scaffold

In vitro
culture

In vivo model for long bone

In mice

Clinical Study

Fig. 8.6 Experimental model

The approach for the use of MSCs-based implants of bone cells to enhance bone repair will eliminate the need for additional surgical procedure, reduce unnecessary pain and complications to the patient, and shorten hospitalization time. The stromal compartment of the cavities of bone is composed of a net-like structure of interconnected MSCs. Stromal cells are closely associated with bone cortex, bone trabecules, and the hematopoietic cells. The MSCs-derived osteoprogenitor cells can be used in modern technology for tissue engineering and cell therapy. They can be used in metabolic bone diseases and orthopedic approaches, when bone repair is needed. By accomplishing the task of identifying of specific osteoprogenitors, the selection of osteoprogenitor cells from the bone marrow will be available [9, 121] (Fig. 8.3). The hypothesis is that osteoprogenitor cells derived from MSCs implanted in a biological scaffold can enhance the repair of bone defects, and will accelerate fracture healing specially in aging and bone disease. These cells are under the effects of growth factors and the 3D supporting microenvironment of the bone marrow. It has been reported that supplementation of bone marrow stromal cells cultures with FGF-2 resulted in prolonged lifespan of bone marrow stromal cells to more than 70 doublings and maintained their differentiation potential accompanied by an increase of their telomerase size [122]. MSCs from adult bone marrow are multipotent cells which can differentiate into fibroblastic, osteogenic, myogenic, adipogenic, and reticular cells. These cells may also provide a potential therapy for bone repair.

These selected cells were shown to produce a bone-specific matrix that was positive for osteocalcin. The matrix synthesized by the selected osteoprogenitors also stained positively with Alizarin Red S and von Kossa indicating both the synthesis of bone primary osteoid matrix and the subsequent mineralization of the matrix. Osteoprogenitors derived from MSCs were shown to express specific bone markers at various stages of the culture. Osteogenic differentiation stages could be divided into three periods that coincide with days in culture. The development of an osteo-conductive slow-release device containing committed bone forming bone cells and growth factors will minimize the need for autologous bone grafts used today for filling bone voids or gaps and will thereby reduce the inherent risks and complications associated with the additional surgery of bone harvesting. Reinforcing the developed osteogenic bone graft substitute will improve the mechanical properties of the device, thereby extending its potential applications to highly loaded locations in the human body. Introduction of such bone substitute into clinical practice will restore the mobility and improve the quality of life of both young and aging patients who lost bone during trauma or surgical resection. One of the technical problems in conducting in vivo experiments on rat is the difficulty to aspirate a bone marrow without scarifying the animal, and for that reason preliminary in vivo results were not introduced. To solve this obstacle, larger animal such as rabbit was used. In rabbits it was possible to aspirate bone marrow and to culture it on the hydrogel, our primarily results on mandible defect revealed bone regeneration in critical size defect. It is hypothesized that growth factors and selected bone forming cells that will be incorporated in osteoinductive osteoconductive scaffolds will enhance bone formation. The hydrogel with appropriate biodegradability will function not only as a release matrix for the growth factors and supporting MSCs, but also as a space provided for bone osseointegration affecting the firmness of the fixation implants. The hydrogel containing growth factors and bone forming cells is thus a promising surgical tool for bone defects and for orthopedic and maxillofacial surgery.

References

1. D'Ippolito G, Schiller PC, Ricordi C, Roos BA, Howard GA (1999) Age-related osteogenic potential of mesenchymal stromal stem cells from human vertebral bone marrow. J Bone Miner Res 14:1115–1122
2. Owen M, Friedenstein AJ (1988) Stromal stem cells: marrow-derived osteogenic precursors. Ciba Found Symp 136:42–60
3. Hasegawa S, Tamura J, Neo M, Goto K, Shikinami Y, Saito M, Kita M, Nakamura T (2005) In vivo evaluation of a porous hydroxyapatite/poly-DL-lactide composite for use as a bone substitute. J Biomed Mater Res A 75:567–579
4. Srouji S, Kizhner T, Livne E (2006) 3D scaffolds for bone marrow stem cell support in bone repair. Regen Med 1:519–528
5. Srouji S, Kizhner T, Suss-Tobi E, Livne E, Zussman E (2008) 3-D Nanofibrous electrospun multilayered construct is an alternative ECM mimicking scaffold. J Mater Sci Mater Med 19:1249–1255
6. Khan Y, Yaszemski MJ, Mikos AG, Laurencin CT (2008) Tissue engineering of bone: material and matrix considerations. J Bone Joint Surg Am 90(Suppl 1):36–42

7. Schaefer D, Martin I, Jundt G, Seidel J, Heberer M, Grodzinsky A, Bergin I, Vunjak-Novakovic G, Freed LE (2002) Tissue-engineered composites for the repair of large osteochondral defects. Arthritis Rheum 46:2524–2534
8. Service RF (2000) Tissue engineers build new bone. Science 289:1498–1500
9. Bianco P, Riminucci M, Gronthos S, Robey PG (2001) Bone marrow stromal stem cells: nature, biology, and potential applications. Stem Cells 19:180–192
10. Bianco P, Robey PG (2001) Stem cells in tissue engineering. Nature 414:118–121
11. Fialkov JA, Holy CE, Shoichet MS, Davies JE (2003) In vivo bone engineering in a rabbit femur. J Craniofac Surg 14:324–332
12. Quarto R, Mastrogiacomo M, Cancedda R, Kutepov SM, Mukhachev V, Lavroukov A, Kon E, Marcacci M (2001) Repair of large bone defects with the use of autologous bone marrow stromal cells. N Engl J Med 344:385–386
13. Fleming JE Jr, Cornell CN, Muschler GF (2000) Bone cells and matrices in orthopedic tissue engineering. Orthop Clin North Am 31:357–374
14. Robey PG (2000) Stem cells near the century mark. J Clin Invest 105:1489–1491
15. Robey PG, Kuznetsov SA, Riminucci M, Bianco P (2007) Skeletal ("mesenchymal") stem cells for tissue engineering. Methods Mol Med 140:83–99
16. Srouji S, Livne E (2005) Bone marrow stem cells and biological scaffold for bone repair in aging and disease. Mech Ageing Dev 126:281–287
17. Martin TJ, Ng KW, Nicholson GC (1988) Cell biology of bone. Baillieres Clin Endocrinol Metab 2:1–29
18. Hynes RO (1992) Integrins: versatility, modulation, and signaling in cell adhesion. Cell 69:11–25
19. Mohan S, Baylink DJ (1991) Bone growth factors. Clin Orthop 263:30–48
20. Lind M (1996) Growth factors: possible new clinical tools. A review. Acta Orthop Scand 67:407–417
21. Lind M, Overgaard S, Ongpipattanakul B, Nguyen T, Bunger C, Soballe K (1996) Transforming growth factor-beta 1 stimulates bone ongrowth to weight-loaded tricalcium phosphate coated implants: an experimental study in dogs. J Bone Joint Surg Br 78:377–382
22. Urist MR (1965) Bone: formation by autoinduction. Science 150:893–899
23. Urist MR, Strates BS (1971) Bone morphogenetic protein. J Dent Res 50:1392–1406
24. Duguy N, Petite H, Arnaud E (2000) Biomaterials and osseous regeneration. Ann Chir Plast Esthet 45:364–376
25. Groeneveld EH, Burger EH (2000) Bone morphogenetic proteins in human bone regeneration. Eur J Endocrinol 142:9–21
26. Asahina I, Sampath TK, Nishimura I, Hauschka PV (1993) Human osteogenic protein-1 induces both chondroblastic and osteoblastic differentiation of osteoprogenitor cells derived from newborn rat calvaria. J Cell Biol 123:921–933
27. Hughes FJ, Collyer J, Stanfield M, Goodman SA (1995) The effects of bone morphogenetic protein-2, -4, and -6 on differentiation of rat osteoblast cells in vitro. Endocrinology 136:2671–2677
28. Okubo Y, Bessho K, Fujimura K, Iizuka T, Miyatake S (1999) Expression of bone morphogenetic protein-2 via adenoviral vector in C2C12 myoblasts induces differentiation into the osteoblast lineage. Biochem Biophys Res Commun 262:739–743
29. Takita H, Vehof JW, Jansen JA, Yamamoto M, Tabata Y, Tamura M, Kuboki Y (2004) Carrier dependent cell differentiation of bone morphogenetic protein-2 induced osteogenesis and chondrogenesis during the early implantation stage in rats. J Biomed Mater Res A 71:181–189
30. Bonewald LF, Mundy GR (1990) Role of transforming growth factor-beta in bone remodeling. Clin Orthop 250:261–276
31. Nielsen HM, Andreassen TT, Ledet T, Oxlund H (1994) Local injection of TGF-beta increases the strength of tibial fractures in the rat. Acta Orthop Scand 65:37–41
32. Lind M, Schumacker B, Soballe K, Keller J, Melsen F, Bunger C (1993) Transforming growth factor-beta enhances fracture healing in rabbit tibiae. Acta Orthop Scand 64:553–556
33. Sonntag WE, Steger RW, Forman LJ, Meites J (1980) Decreased pulsatile release of growth hormone in old male rats. Endocrinology 107:1875–1879

34. Radomsky ML,Thompson AY, Spiro RC, Poser JW (1998) Potential role of fibroblast growth factor in enhancement of fracture healing. Clin Orthop 350:S283–S293
35. Yao W, Hadi T, Jiang Y, Lotz J, Wronski TJ, Lane NE (2005) Basic fibroblast growth factor improves trabecular bone connectivity and bone strength in the lumbar vertebral body of osteopenic rats. Osteoporos Int 16:1939–1947
36. Nakamura K, Kurokawa T, Aoyama I, Hanada K, Tamura M, Kawaguchi H (1998) Stimulation of bone formation by intraosseous injection of basic fibroblast growth factor in ovariectomised rats. Int Orthop 22:49–54
37. Ichinohe N, Kuboki Y, Tabata Y (2008) Bone regeneration using titanium nonwoven fabrics combined with fgf-2 release from gelatin hydrogel microspheres in rabbit skull defects. Tissue Eng Part A 14:1663–1671
38. Wozney JM, Rosen V, Celeste AJ, Mitsock LM, Whitters MJ, Kriz RW, Hewick RM, Wang EA (1988) Novel regulators of bone formation: molecular clones and activities. Science 242:1528–1534
39. Hulth A (1989) Current concepts of fracture healing. Clin Orthop 249:265–284
40. Sandberg MM, Aro HT, Vuorio EI (1993) Gene expression during bone repair. Clin Orthop 289:292–312
41. Centrella M, McCarthy TL, Canalis E (1987) Transforming growth factor beta is a bifunctional regulator of replication and collagen synthesis in osteoblast-enriched cell cultures from fetal rat bone. J Biol Chem 262:2869–2874
42. Centrella M, McCarthy TL, Canalis E (1987) Mitogenesis in fetal rat bone cells simultaneously exposed to type beta transforming growth factor and other growth regulators. FASEB J 1:312–317
43. Robey PG, Young MF, Flanders KC, Roche NS, Kondaiah P, Reddi AH, Termine JD, Sporn MB, Roberts AB (1987) Osteoblasts synthesize and respond to transforming growth factor-type beta (TGF-beta) in vitro. J Cell Biol 105:457–463
44. Lucas PA (1989) Chemotactic response of osteoblast-like cells to transforming growth factor beta. Bone 10:459–463
45. Blumenfeld, I., Srouji, S., Lanir, Y., Laufer, D. & Livne, E. (2002) Enhancement of bone defect healing in old rats by tgf-beta and igf-1. Exp Gerontol 37: 553–565
46. Blumenfeld, I., Srouji, S., Peled, M. & Livne, E. (2002) Metalloproteinases (mmps -2, -3) are involved in tgf-beta and igf-1-induced bone defect healing in 20-month-old female rats. Arch Gerontol Geriatr 35: 59–69
47. Augat P, Margevicius K, Simon J, Wolf S, Suger G, Claes L (1998) Local tissue properties in bone healing: influence of size and stability of the osteotomy gap. J Orthop Res 16: 475–481
48. Srouji S, Rachmiel A, Blumenfeld I, Livne E (2005) Mandibular defect repair by TGF-beta and IGF-1 released from a biodegradable osteoconductive hydrogel. J Craniomaxillofac Surg 33:79–84
49. Srouji S, Blumenfeld I, Rachmiel A, Livne E (2004) Bone defect repair in rat tibia by TGF-beta1 and IGF-1 released from hydrogel scaffold. Cell Tissue Bank 5:223–230
50. Ettinger MP (2003) Aging bone and osteoporosis: strategies for preventing fractures in the elderly. Arch Intern Med 163:2237–2246
51. Seeman E (2003) The structural and biomechanical basis of the gain and loss of bone strength in women and men. Endocrinol Metab Clin North Am 32:25–38
52. Schmitz JP, Hollinger JO (1986) The critical size defect as an experimental model for craniomandibulofacial nonunions. Clin Orthop 205:299–308
53. Robey PG, Bianco P (2006) The use of adult stem cells in rebuilding the human face. J Am Dent Assoc 137:961–972
54. Benayahu D (2000) The hematopoietic microenvironment: the osteogenic compartment of bone marrow: cell biology and clinical application. Hematology 4:427–435
55. Benayahu D, Fried A, Efraty M, Robey PG, Wientroub S (1995) Bone marrow interface: preferential attachment of an osteoblastic marrow stromal cell line. J Cell Biochem 59:151–160

56. D'Ippolito G, Romano G, Caruso T, Spinella A, Cimino G, Fontana A (2003) Production of octadienal in the marine diatom *Skeletonema costatum*. Org Lett 5:885–887

57. Bianco P, Robey PG, Simmons PJ (2008) Mesenchymal stem cells: revisiting history, concepts, and assays. Cell Stem Cell 2:313–319

58. Beresford JN (1989) Osteogenic stem cells and the stromal system of bone and marrow. Clin Orthop 240:270–280

59. Cheng SL, Yang JW, Rifas L, Zhang SF, Avioli LV (1994) Differentiation of human bone marrow osteogenic stromal cells in vitro: induction of the osteoblast phenotype by dexamethasone. Endocrinology 134:277–286

60. Herbertson A, Aubin JE (1995) Dexamethasone alters the subpopulation make-up of rat bone marrow stromal cell cultures. J Bone Miner Res 10:285–294

61. Barrilleaux B, Phinney DG, Prockop DJ, O'Connor KC (2006) Review: ex vivo engineering of living tissues with adult stem cells. Tissue Eng 12:3007–3019

62. Shalhoub V, Conlon D, Tassinari M, Quinn C, Partridge N, Stein GS, Lian JB (1992) Glucocorticoids promote development of the osteoblast phenotype by selectively modulating expression of cell growth and differentiation associated genes. J Cell Biochem 50:425–440

63. Maniatopoulos C, Sodek J, Melcher AH (1988) Bone formation in vitro by stromal cells obtained from bone marrow of young adult rats. Cell Tissue Res 254:317–330

64. Bellows CG, Heersche JN, Aubin JE (1990) Determination of the capacity for proliferation and differentiation of osteoprogenitor cells in the presence and absence of dexamethasone. Dev Biol 140:132–138

65. Lian JB, Stein GS (1992) Concepts of osteoblast growth and differentiation: basis for modulation of bone cell development and tissue formation. Crit Rev Oral Biol Med 3:269–305

66. Leblond CP (1964) Classification of cell populations on the basis of their proliferative behavior. Natl Cancer Inst Monogr 14:119–150

67. Weissman IL (2000) Stem cells: units of development, units of regeneration, and units in evolution. Cell 100:157–168

68. Mankani MH, Kuznetsov SA, Robey PG (2007) Formation of hematopoietic territories and bone by transplanted human bone marrow stromal cells requires a critical cell density. Exp Hematol 35:995–1004

69. Friedenstein AJ, Piatetzky S II, Petrakova KV (1966) Osteogenesis in transplants of bone marrow cells. J Embryol Exp Morphol 16:381–390

70. Pittenger MF, Mosca JD, McIntosh KR (2000) Human mesenchymal stem cells: progenitor cells for cartilage, bone, fat and stroma. Curr Top Microbiol Immunol 251:3–11

71. McKay R (2000) Stem cells–hype and hope. Nature 406:361–364

72. Hayashi K, Kubo T, Doi K, Tabata Y, Akagawa Y (2007) Development of new drug delivery system for implant bone augmentation using a basic fibroblast growth factor-gelatin hydrogel complex. Dent Mater J 26:170–177

73. Van Vlierberghe S, Cnudde V, Masschaele B, Dubruel P, De Paepe I, Jacobs PJ, Van Hoorebeke L, Unger R, Kirkpatrick CJ, Schacht EH (2006) Porous gelatin cryogels as cell delivery tool in tissue engineering. J Control Release 116:e95–e98

74. Chong EJ, Phan TT, Lim IJ, Zhang YZ, Bay BH, Ramakrishna S, Lim CT (2007) Evaluation of electrospun PCL/gelatin nanofibrous scaffold for wound healing and layered dermal reconstitution. Acta Biomater 3:321–330

75. Fedorovich NE, De Wijn JR, Verbout AJ, Alblas J, Dhert WJ (2008) Three-dimensional fiber deposition of cell-laden, viable, patterned constructs for bone tissue printing. Tissue Eng Part A 14:127–133

76. Lee SC, Shea M, Battle MA, Kozitza K, Ron E, Turek T, Schaub RG, Hayes WC (1994) Healing of large segmental defects in rat femurs is aided by RhBMP-2 in PLGA matrix. J Biomed Mater Res 28:1149–1156

77. Ueki K, Takazakura D, Marukawa K, Shimada M, Nakagawa K, Takatsuka S, Yamamoto E (2003) The use of polylactic acid/polyglycolic acid copolymer and gelatin sponge complex containing human recombinant bone morphogenetic protein-2 following condylectomy in rabbits. J Craniomaxillofac Surg 31:107–114

78. Higuchi T, Kinoshita A, Takahashi K, Oda S, Ishikawa I (1999) Bone regeneration by recombinant human bone morphogenetic protein-2 in rat mandibular defects. An experimental model of defect filling. J Periodontol 70:1026–1031

79. Lind M, Overgaard S, Soballe K, Nguyen T, Ongpipattanakul B, Bunger C (1996) Transforming growth factor-beta 1 enhances bone healing to unloaded tricalcium phosphate coated implants: an experimental study in dogs. J Orthop Res 14:343–350

80. Bell R, Beirne OR (1988) Effect of hydroxylapatite, tricalcium phosphate, and collagen on the healing of defects in the rat mandible. J Oral Maxillofac Surg 46:589–594

81. Bohner M (2000) Calcium orthophosphates in medicine: from ceramics to calcium phosphate cements. Injury 31(Suppl 4):37–47

82. Bohner M, Lemaitre J, Merkle HP, Gander B (2000) Control of gentamicin release from a calcium phosphate cement by admixed poly(acrylic acid). J Pharm Sci 89:1262–1270

83. Saito A, Suzuki Y, Kitamura M, Ogata S, Yoshihara Y, Masuda S, Ohtsuki C, Tanihara M (2006) Repair of 20-mm long rabbit radial bone defects using BMP-derived peptide combined with an alpha-tricalcium phosphate scaffold. J Biomed Mater Res A 77:700–706

84. Stubbs D, Deakin M, Chapman-Sheath P, Bruce W, Debes J, Gillies RM, Walsh WR (2004) In vivo evaluation of resorbable bone graft substitutes in a rabbit tibial defect model. Biomaterials 25:5037–5044

85. Livingston T, Ducheyne P, Garino J (2002) In vivo evaluation of a bioactive scaffold for bone tissue engineering. J Biomed Mater Res 62:1–13

86. Yamamoto M, Ikada Y, Tabata Y (2001) Controlled release of growth factors based on bio-degradation of gelatin hydrogel. J Biomater Sci Polym Ed 12:77–88

87. Yamamoto M, Sakakibara Y, Nishimura K, Komeda M, Tabata Y (2003) Improved therapeutic efficacy in cardiomyocyte transplantation for myocardial infarction with release system of basic fibroblast growth factor. Artif Organs 27:181–184

88. Yamamoto M, Tabata Y, Hong L, Miyamoto S, Hashimoto N, Ikada Y (2000) Bone regeneration by transforming growth factor beta1 released from a biodegradable hydrogel. J Control Release 64:133–142

89. Fedorovich NE, Alblas J, de Wijn JR, Hennink WE, Verbout AJ, Dhert WJ (2007) Hydrogels as extracellular matrices for skeletal tissue engineering: state-of-the-art and novel application in organ printing. Tissue Eng 13:1905–1925

90. Dubruel P, Unger R, Vlierberghe SV, Cnudde V, Jacobs PJ, Schacht E, Kirkpatrick CJ (2007) Porous gelatin hydrogels: 2 In vitro cell interaction study. Biomacromolecules 8:338–344

91. Park H, Temenoff JS, Tabata Y, Caplan AI, Mikos AG (2007) Injectable biodegradable hydrogel composites for rabbit marrow mesenchymal stem cell and growth factor delivery for cartilage tissue engineering. Biomaterials 28:3217–3227

92. Hasegawa S, Ishii S, Tamura J, Furukawa T, Neo M, Matsusue Y, Shikinami Y, Okuno M, Nakamura T (2006) A 5-7 year in vivo study of high-strength hydroxyapatite/poly(L-lactide) composite rods for the internal fixation of bone fractures. Biomaterials 27:1327–1332

93. Walsh WR, Harrison J, Loefler A, Martin T, Van Sickle D, Brown MK, Sonnabend DH (2000) Mechanical and histologic evaluation of collagraft in an ovine lumbar fusion model. Clin Orthop 375:258–66

94. Rodan GA, Martin TJ (2000) Therapeutic approaches to bone diseases. Science 289:1508–1514

95. Sikavitsas VI, Temenoff JS, Mikos AG (2001) Biomaterials and bone mechanotransduction. Biomaterials 22:2581–2593

96. Franceschi RT, Xiao G (2003) Regulation of the osteoblast-specific transcription factor, Runx2: responsiveness to multiple signal transduction pathways. J Cell Biochem 88:446–454

97. Botchwey EA, Pollack SR, Levine EM, Laurencin CT (2001) Bone tissue engineering in a rotating bioreactor using a microcarrier matrix system. J Biomed Mater Res 55:242–253

98. Tabata Y, Yamada K, Miyamoto S, Nagata I, Kikuchi H, Aoyama I, Tamura M, Ikada Y (1998) Bone regeneration by basic fibroblast growth factor complexed with biodegradable hydrogels. Biomaterials 19:807–815

99. Trantolo DJ, Sonis ST, Thompson BM, Wise DL, Lewandrowski KU, Hile DD (2003) Evaluation of a porous, biodegradable biopolymer scaffold for mandibular reconstruction. Int J Oral Maxillofac Implants 18:182–188

100. Bosch C, Melsen B, Gibbons R, Vargervik K (1996) Human recombinant transforming growth factor-beta 1 in healing of calvarial bone defects. J Craniofac Surg 7:300–310

101. Sherris DA, Murakami CS, Larrabee WF Jr, Bruce AG (1998) Mandibular reconstruction with transforming growth factor-beta1. Laryngoscope 108:368–372

102. Zambonin G, Losito I, Triffitt JT, Zambonin CG (2000) Detection of collagen synthesis by human osteoblasts on a tricalcium phosphate hydroxyapatite: an X-ray photoelectron spectroscopy investigation. J Biomed Mater Res 49:120–126

103. Blumenfeld I, Srouji S, Peled M, Livne E (2002) Metalloproteinases (MMPs -2, -3) are involved in TGF-beta and IGF-1-induced bone defect healing in 20-month-old female rats. Arch Gerontol Geriatr 35:59–69

104. Bruder SP, Jaiswal N, Ricalton NS, Mosca JD, Kraus KH, Kadiyala S (1998) Mesenchymal stem cells in osteobiology and applied bone regeneration. Clin Orthop 355:S247–S256

105. Bruder SP, Kurth AA, Shea M, Hayes WC, Jaiswal N, Kadiyala S (1998) Bone regeneration by implantation of purified, culture-expanded human mesenchymal stem cells. J Orthop Res 16:155–162

106. Gombotz WR, Pankey SC, Bouchard LS, Phan DH, Puolakkainen PA (1994) Stimulation of bone healing by transforming growth factor-beta 1 released from polymeric or ceramic implants. J Appl Biomater 5:141–150

107. Moxham JP, Kibblewhite DJ, Bruce AG, Rigley T, Gillespy T 3rd, Lane J (1996) Transforming growth factor-beta 1 in a guanidine-extracted demineralized bone matrix carrier rapidly closes a rabbit critical calvarial defect. J Otolaryngol 25:82–87

108. Hutmacher DW (2000) Scaffolds in tissue engineering bone and cartilage. Biomaterials 21:2529–2543

109. Toung JS, Griffin A, Ogle RC, Lindsey WH (1998) Repair of nasal defects using collagen gels containing insulin-like growth factor 1. Laryngoscope 108:1654–1658

110. Hong L, Tabata Y, Yamamoto M, Miyamoto S, Yamada K, Hashimoto N, Ikada Y (1998) Comparison of bone regeneration in a rabbit skull defect by recombinant human BMP-2 incorporated in biodegradable hydrogel and in solution. J Biomater Sci Polym Ed 9:1001–1014

111. Lindsey WH, Franz DA, Toung JS, London SD, Ogle RO (1998) A nasal critical-size defect: an experimental model for the evaluation of facial osseous repair techniques. Arch Otolaryngol Head Neck Surg 124:912–915

112. Van Vlierberghe S, Dubruel P, Lippens E, Masschaele B, Van Hoorebeke L, Cornelissen M, Unger R, Kirkpatrick CJ, Schacht E (2008) Toward modulating the architecture of hydrogel scaffolds: curtains versus channels. J Mater Sci Mater Med 19:1459–1466

113. Vermonden T, Fedorovich NE, van Geemen D, Alblas J, van Nostrum CF, Dhert WJ, Hennink WE (2008) Photopolymerized thermosensitive hydrogels: synthesis, degradation, and cytocompatibility. Biomacromolecules 9:919–926

114. Fedorovich NE, Oudshoorn MH, van Geemen D, Hennink WE, Alblas J, Dhert WJ (2009) The effect of photopolymerization on stem cells embedded in hydrogels. Biomaterials 30:344–353

115. Weizmann S, Tong A, Reich A, Genina O, Yayon A, Monsonego-Ornan E (2005) FGF upregulates osteopontin in epiphyseal growth plate chondrocytes: implications for endochondral ossification. Matrix Biol 24(8):520–529

116. Yang F, Williams CG, Wang DA, Lee H, Manson PN, Elisseeff J (2005) The effect of incorporating RGD adhesive peptide in polyethylene glycol diacrylate hydrogel on osteogenesis of bone marrow stromal cells. Biomaterials 26:5991–5998

117. Sumanasinghe RD, Osborne JA, Loboa EG (2009) Mesenchymal stem cell-seeded collagen matrices for bone repair: effects of cyclic tensile strain, cell density, and media conditions on matrix contraction in vitro. J Biomed Mater Res A 88:778–786

118. Randle WL, Cha JM, Hwang YS, Chan KL, Kazarian SG, Polak JM, Mantalaris A (2007) Integrated 3-dimensional expansion and osteogenic differentiation of murine embryonic stem cells. Tissue Eng 13:2957–2970

119. Tatebe M, Nakamura R, Kagami H, Okada K, Ueda M (2005) Differentiation of transplanted mesenchymal stem cells in a large osteochondral defect in rabbit. Cytotherapy 7:520–530
120. Hollinger JO, Kleinschmidt JC (1990) The critical size defect as an experimental model to test bone repair materials. J Craniofac Surg 1:60–68
121. Bianco P, Gehron Robey P (2000) Marrow stromal stem cells. J Clin Invest 105:1663–1668
122. Bianchi G, Banfi A, Mastrogiacomo M, Notaro R, Luzzatto L, Cancedda R, Quarto R (2003) Ex vivo enrichment of mesenchymal cell progenitors by fibroblast growth factor 2. Exp Cell Res 287:98–105

Chapter 9
Bone Reaction to Implants

David Kohavi

9.1 Introduction

Endosseous insertion of an artificial orthopedic or dental material induces an extensive tissue reaction at the implant–bone interface. Formation of a bone–implant attachment has been regularly reported. Bone repair in these instances is portrayed in several patterns. Healing depends on systemic and local conditions, inter alia, bone status, surgical technique, implant surface, biomechanical properties, and forces used. Osseointegration is defined as a direct structural bonding between bone tissue and implant surface. Clinically, such implant attachment produces a firm, asymptomatic fixation maintained in bone under functional loading. In other instances, healing is completed by fibro-integration, namely, implants are surrounded by fibrous connective tissue, showing an evident clinical mobility when loaded [1–6]. In osseointegration, light microscopy (LM) reveals insignificant amounts of fibrous tissue at the bone–implant interface; all in all, bone formation is characterized by attachment to the largest part of implant surface. Utilization of titanium alloy (Ti) implants revealed an optimal capability for osseointegration. Consequently, Ti is considered material of choice in orthopedic and oral implants. Additionally, this has been supported by biomechanical studies that showed insignificant mobility of Ti implants [7–10]. Implant stability is affected by biomechanical properties of the adjacent bone. Cortical bone allows a more stable mechanical anchorage of the implant than trabecular bone [8, 11]. Structural and mechanical changes due to impaired bone may well be responsible for reduced stability of implants [12]. Different surgical techniques have shown a significant effect on implant fixation in trabecular bone [13]. A close contact between implant and bone

D. Kohavi (✉)
Institute of Dental Sciences, The Hebrew University Hadassah –
Faculty of Dental Medicine, P.O. Box 12272, Jerusalem, 91120, Israel
e-mail: kohavi@cc.huji.ac.il

J.J. Sela and I.A. Bab (eds.), *Principles of Bone Regeneration*,
DOI 10.1007/978-1-4614-2059-0_9, © Springer Science+Business Media, LLC 2012

does not necessarily serve to enhance osteogenesis. On the other hand, wide space of more than 500 μm is predictive of delay and reduction in the quality or quantity of the newly formed bone [14–20]. Excessive load on the implant may enhance fibrous membrane formation and displacement at the bone–implant interface preventing osseointegration [21–26]. The principal mechanisms essential for osseointegration could be compared to those occurring in fracture repair and involve a cascade of various cellular and extracellular events [22]. The insertion of an implant is in effect an excision-injury within bone tissue, often accompanied by an increase in temperature [23]. Surgical procedure is followed by blood clotting and inflammatory reaction at implant surface. Cellular infiltrate consists of polymorphonuclear granulocytes, monocytes, macrophages, osteoclasts, and osteoblasts that migrate into the tissue adjacent to the implant. The implant surface adsorbs blood-derived proteins [24–26]. Exposure of Ti implants to plasma is followed by an immediate coating of its surface by a thin proteinaceous film. Albumin, fibronectin, fibrinogen, and IgG are the main constituents [27–30]. The extent of plasma protein adsorption to the surface is an essential indicator for implant biocompatibility [28]. Cellular attachment to biomaterial surface ensues following the interaction of adsorbed soluble proteins to cell-surface-integrins. The protein type and amount may affect cellular proliferation, differentiation, and migration [29]. Increased levels of plasma fibronectin (pFN), a high molecular weight extracellular matrix glycoprotein, are evident in early phases of cell growth and attachment [30, 31]. In osteoblast regulation, pFN activates signaling pathways of gene expression, cell-cycle progression, matrix mineralization, and apoptosis [32, 33]. Plasma protein adhesion to implants and the interaction with blood cells are required for osteoconduction [34]. Biomaterial surfaces coated by pFN showed an enhanced focal adhesion of osteoclasts, essential to improve cell spreading and cytoskeleton organization as compared to non-coated surfaces [35–39]. Serum albumin, constituting circa 60% of human plasma protein, serves as a carrier for molecules of low water solubility, including various hormones and ionic calcium. Albumin-bound lipids regulate cytoplasm calcium levels and stimulate osteoblast proliferation [40]. Protein adsorption is dependent on implant surface chemistry, structure, and morphology [41–43]. It has been shown that cell attachment and proliferation are surface roughness sensitive. Ergo, surface modifications of titanium are of main interest in the study of osteoconductivity of implants [44]. Protein adsorption appears to be roughness-dependent and human serum albumin is preferentially adsorbed on the smooth Ti surfaces, while fibronectin and total protein manifest increased binding to rough Ti surfaces. On surfaces with rough micro-topographies, osteoblasts were shown to secrete factors that enhance their differentiation and decrease osteoclasts formation and activation [45]. Nano-texturing of Ti surfaces offers an improved cell attachment, influencing cell density and morphology and regulating early expression of bone proteins [46, 47]. Confocal microscope studies revealed a significantly higher amount of albumin on the acid-etched and blasted surfaces as compared to machined and acid-etched surfaces [35]. The early cellular response to Ti implants involves deposition of non-collagenous layer on the implant surface by osteogenic cells. This is similar to the observation of bone cement lines and lamina limitans [33, 48–50].

Morphological studies reported heterogeneity in implant–bone interface. However, the early non-fibrillar, calcified layer presented a high similarity in all implants despite the different type of surfaces. Migration of mesenchymal stem cells (MSCs) is followed by colonization of the implant surface. MSCs differentiate into osteoblasts that secrete a 0.5-μm-thick fibrous collagen layer. Ionic calcium and phosphorus regulate cell adhesion and mineralization, resulting with new bone formation on the implant surface [51–54]. The interaction of red blood cells, fibrin, and platelets with the implant surface may modulate migration and differentiation [55]. Osteoblast and osteoclast activity is observed at the implant surface from day 1 of insertion [56–61]. Newly formed bone at the Interface of the surgically created implant cavity shows high similarity to the one observed in bone wound healing. The mineralized matrix is subject to resorption by osteoclasts. "Cement lines" implicated in cellular attachment, 0.2–5-μm wide, are composed sulfated polysaccharide complexes and osteopontin demarcate the transition between bone resorption formation [33, 57–61]. Cement lines at bone implant interface bear resemblance to analogous ones detected in bone remodeling [33]. On the first week of implantation, osteoblasts deposit collagen matrix directly on cement line formed on implant surface [33, 49, 61–65]. The early deposition of new calcified matrix on the implant surface is followed by formation of woven spongiosa and mature lamellar trabecular bone [23, 24]. Bone marrow provides mononuclear precursors of osteoclasts for trabecular remodeling [65]. Woven bone formation occurs on the implant surface and establishes initial continuity, albeit poor mechanical competence [66]. Remodeling of primary young bone allows its replacement by highly mineralized lamellar and trabecular bone with improved biomechanical properties. Mature bone has been found around different types of Ti implants 3 months after implantation [66, 67]. Two orientations of bone formation were observed at the implant interface, toward the implant surface and starting at the implant surface [65]. Vascular disruption and osteoclast activity are implicated in implant separation. [67, 68]. In osseointegration of metallic implants, bone healing did not start on the implant surface, and bone was shown to develop toward the implant [51, 69–73]. Changes at the titanium–bone interface have been detected with LM, transmission electron microscopy (TEM), and micro-computed tomography (μCT). These showed that Ti implants induced an immediate cellular alignment on bone and implant surfaces. On day 14, new bone was found in direct contact with the implant. TEM images showed flat osteoblasts with rich rough endoplasmic reticulum along the surfaces of the implant and the preexisting bone secreting collagen and beginning of calcification. μCT images on day 13 after implant insertion showed new bone formation. Surface roughness of titanium implants affects various determinants of osseointegration such as protein adsorption, osteoblast attachment and subsequent proliferation and differentiation, extracellular matrix production, alkaline phosphatase activity, periimplant bone formation, and primary implant stability. Roughness may also influence two local factors, TGFb1 and PGE2, acting as autocrine regulators on the osteoblasts and modulating the activity of osteoclasts [74–76]. It has been suggested that the roughness-dependent regulation of osteoblast proliferation, differentiation, and production of local factors is mediated by integrin receptors that regulate phosphokinase C (PKC) and A (PKA) through phospholipase C (PLC) and A2 (PLA2) pathways [77]. Generally, at the micrometer grade level of evaluation, moderately rough surfaces favor peri-implant bone growth better than smoother or rougher surfaces [78–81].

Coating of titanium implant surface with hydroxyapatite (HA) or other calcium phosphate compounds may accelerate peri-implant osteogenesis and provide a mechanical barrier to metal ion release or titanium particles detachment [82–86]. Glass-ceramic coating was shown to increase implant bonding, and it was suggested that newly formed collagen tends to attach to the chemically active surface of these biomimetic materials [87]. Bone formation increases at beta-tricalcium phosphate (TCP) cylinders when compared to HA ceramics with the same pore size. Among different pore sizes, a pore size above 80 μm has been shown to improve bone attachment in both HA and TCP materials. HA-coated implants showed earlier bone formation when compared to titanium surfaces as tested by removal torque tests and histomorphometric analyze [88–90]. In addition rough surfaces increase interface contact area contributing to implant primary stability [91–93].

References

1. Brånemark PI, Adell R, Breine U, Hansson BO, Lindström J, Ohlsson A (1969) Intra-osseous anchorage of dental prostheses. I. Experimental studies. Scand J Plast Reconstr Surg 3(2):81–100
2. Albrektsson T, Branemark P-I, Hansson H-A, Lindström J (1981) Osseointegrated titanium implants. Requirements for ensuring a long-lasting, direct bone-to implant anchorage in man. Acta Orthop Scand 52:155–170
3. Branemark PI (1985) Introduction to osseointegration. In: Branemark P-I, Zarb GA, Albrektsson T (eds) Tissue integrated prostheses. Quintessence Publishing, Chicago, pp 11–76
4. Steinemann SG, Eulenberger J, Maeusll PA, Schroeder A (1989) Adhesion of bone to titanium. In: Christel P, Meunier A, Lee AJC (eds) Biological and biomechanical performance of biomaterials. Elsevier, Amsterdam, pp 409–414
5. Zarb GA, Albrektsson T (1991) Osseointegration: a requiem for the periodontal ligament? Int J Periodont Rest Dent 11:88–91
6. Natiella JR, Armitage JE, Meenaghan MA, Greene GW (1974) Tissue response to dental implants protruding through mucous membrane. Oral Sci Rev 5:85–105
7. Esposito M, Hirsch J-M, Lekholm U, Thomsen P (1998) Biological factors contributing to failures of osseointegrated oral implants (I) Success criteria and epidemiology. Eur J Oral Sci 106:527–551
8. Adell R, Lekholm U, Rockler B, Branemark PI (1981) 15-year study of osseo-integrated implants in the treatment of the edentulous jaw. Int J Oral Surg 10:387–416
9. Nevins M, Langer B (1993) The successful application of osseointegrated implants to the posterior jaw: a long-term retrospective study. Int J Oral Maxillofac Implants 8:423–428
10. Branemark PI, Hansson BO, Adell R, Breine U, Lindstrom J, Hallen J (1977) Osseointegrated implants in the treatment of the edentulous jaw. Experience from a 10-year period. Scand J Plast Reconstr Surg 16:1–132
11. Lazzara R, Siddiqui AA, Binon P, Feldman SA, Weiner R, Philipps R, Gonshor A (1996) Retrospective multicenter analysis of 31 endosseous dental implants placed over a 5 year period. Clin Oral Implants Res 7:73–83
12. Wittenberg RH, Shea M, Swartz BA, Lee SK, White AA, Hayes WC (1991) Importance of bone mineral density in instrumented spine fusions. Spine 16:647–652

13. Shalabi MM, Wolke JG, Jansen JA (2006) The effects of implant surface roughness and surgical technique on implant fixation in an in vitro model. Clin Oral Implants Res 17(2):172–178

14. Berglundh T, Abrahamsson I, Lang NP, Lindhe J (2003) De novo alveolar bone formation adjacent to endosseous implants. A model study in the dog. Clin Oral Implants Res 14:251–262

15. Franchi M, Bacchelli B, Martini D, De Pasquale V, Orsini E, Ottani V, Fini M, Giavaresi G, Giardino R, Ruggeri A (2004) Early detachment of titanium particles from various different surfaces of endosseous dental implants. Biomaterials 25:2239–2246

16. Futami T, Fujii N, Ohnishi H, Taguchi N, Kusakari H, Ohshima H, Maeda T (2000) Tissue response to titanium implants in the rat maxilla: ultrastructural and histochemical observations of the bone titanium interface. J Periodontol 71:287–298

17. Shirakura M, Fujii N, Ohnishi H, Taguchi Y, Ohshima H, Nomura S, Maeda T (2003) Tissue response to titanium implantation in the rat maxilla, with special reference to the effects of surface conditions on bone formation. Clin Oral Implants Res 14:687–696

18. Franchi M, Orsini E, Trire A, Quaranta M, Martini D, Piccari G, Ruggeri A, Ottani V (2004) Osteogenesis and morphology of the peri-implant bone facing dental implants. Scientific World Journal 4:1083–1095

19. Cameron HU, Pilliar RM, Macnab I (1976) The rate of bone ingrowth into porous metal. J Biomed Mater Res 10:259–299

20. Sandborn PM, Cook SD, Spires WP, Kesters MA (1989) Tissue response to porous-coated implants lacking initial bone apposition. J Arthroplasty 3:337–346

21. Carter DR, Giori NJ (1991) In: Davies JE, Albrektsson T (eds) Effect of mechanical stress on tissue differentiation in the bony implant bed, vol 2. University of Toronto Press, Buffalo, pp 367–375

22. Fini M, Giavaresi G, Torricelli P, Corsari V, Giardino R, Nicolini A, Carpi A (2004) Osteoporosis and biomaterial osteointegration. Biomed Pharmacother 58:487–493

23. Listgarten MA (1996) Soft and hard tissue response to endosseous dental implants. Anat Rec 245:410–425

24. Kasemo B, Lausmaa J (1991) The biomaterial-tissue interface and its analogues in surface science and technology. In: Davies JE, Albrektsson T (eds) The bone-biomaterial interface, vol 1. University of Toronto Press, Toronto, pp 19–32

25. Davies JE (1996) In vitro modelling of the bone/implant interface. Anat Rec 245:426–445

26. Park JY, Davies JE (2000) Red blood cell and platelet interactions with titanium implant surfaces. Clin Oral Implants Res 11:530–539

27. Sela MN, Badihi L, Rosen G, Steinberg D, Kohavi D (2007) Adsorption of human plasma proteins to modified titanium surfaces. Clin Oral Implants Res 18(5):630–638, PMID: 17484735

28. Woo KM, Seo J, Zhang R, Ma PX (2007) Suppression of apoptosis by enhanced protein adsorption on polymer/hydroxyapatite composite scaffolds. Biomaterials 28:2622–2630

29. Mata A, Su X, Fleischman AJ, Roy S, Banks BA, Miller SK (2003) Osteoblast attachment to a textured surface in the absence of exogenous adhesion proteins. IEEE Trans Nanobiosci 2:287–294

30. Dean JW 3rd, Culbertson KC, D'Angelo AM (1995) Fibronectin and Laminin enhance gingival cell attachment to dental implant surfaces in vitro. Int J Oral Maxillofac Implants 6:721–728

31. Winnard RG, Gerstenfeld LC, Toma CD, Franceschi RT (1995) Fibronectin gene expression, synthesis and accumulation during in vitro differentiation of chicken osteoblasts. J Bone Miner Res 12:1969–1977

32. Garcia AJ, Reyes CD (2005) Bio-adhesive surfaces to promote osteoblast differentiation and bone formation. J Dent Res 5:407–413

33. Globus RK, Doty SB, Lull JC, Holmuhamedov E, Humphries MJ, Damsky CH (1998) Fibronectin is a survival factor for differentiated osteoblasts. J Cell Sci 111:1385–1393

34. Owens MR, Cimino CD (1982) Synthesis of fibronectin by the isolated perused rat liver. Blood 6:1305–1309

35. Schneider G, Burridge K (1994) Formation of focal adhesions by osteoblasts adhering to different substrata. Exp Cell Res 1:264–269

36. Toworfe GK, Composto RJ, Adams CS, Shapiro IM, Ducheyne P (2004) Fibronectin adsorption on surface-activated poly(dimethylsiloxane) and its effect on cellular function. J Biomed Mater Res A 3:449–461

37. Sauberlich S, Klee D, Richter EJ, Hocker H, Spiekermann H (1999) Cell culture tests for assessing the tolerance of soft tissue to variously modified titanium surfaces. Clin Oral Implants Res 5:379–393

38. Scheideler L, Geis-Gerstorfer J, Kern D, Pfeiffer F, Rupp F, Weber H et al (2003) Investigation of cell reactions to microstructured implant surfaces. Mater Sci Eng C 23:455–459

39. Jimbo R, Sawase T, Shibata Y, Hirata K, Hishikawa Y, Tanaka Y, Bessho K, Ikeda T, Atsuta M (2007) Enhanced Osseointegration by the chemotactic activity of plasma fibronectin for cellular fibronectin positive cells. Biomaterials 28(24):3469–3477

40. Tsai JA, Lagumdzija A, Stark A, Kindmark H (2007) Albumin-bound lipids induce free cytoplasmic calcium oscillations in human osteoblast-like cells. Cell Biochem Funct 25:245–249

41. Yang Y, Dennison D, Ong JL (2005) Protein adsorption and osteoblast precursor cell attachment to hydroxyapatite of different crystallinities. Int J Oral Maxillofac Implants 20:187–192

42. Kern T, Yang Y, Glover R, Ong JL (2005) Effect of heat-treated titanium surfaces on protein adsorption and osteoblast precursor cell initial attachment. Implant Dent 14:70–76

43. Protivinsky J, Appleford M, Strnad J, Helebrant A, Ong JL (2007) Effect of chemically modified titanium surfaces on protein adsorption and osteoblast precursor cell behavior. Int J Oral Maxillofac Implants 22:542–550

44. Deligianni DD, Katsala N, Ladas S, Sotiropoulou D, Amedee J, Missirlis YF (2001) Effect of surface roughness of the titanium alloy Ti–6Al–4V on human bone marrow cell response and on protein adsorption. Biomaterials 22:1241–1251

45. Lossdorfer S, Schwartz Z, Wang L, Lohmann CH, Turner JD, Wieland M, Cochran DL, Boyan BD (2004) Microrough implant surface topographies increase osteogenesis by reducing osteoclast formation and activity. J Biomed Mater Res A 70:361–369

46. Jayaraman M, Meyer U, Buhner M, Joos U, Wiesmann HP (2004) Influence of titanium surfaces on attachment of osteoblast-like cells in vitro. Biomaterials 25:625–631

47. de Oliveira PT, Nanci A (2004) Nanotexturing of titanium-based surfaces up regulates expression of bone sialoprotein and osteopontin by cultured osteogenic cells. Biomaterials 25:403–413

48. Nanci A, McCarthy GF, Zalzal S, Clokie CML, Warshawsky H, McKe MD (1994) Tissue response to titanium implants in the rat tibia: ultrastructural, immunocytochemical and lectin-cytochemical characterization of the bone-titanium interface. Cell Mater 4:1–30

49. Murai K, Takeshita F, Ayukawa Y, Kiyoshima T, Suetsugu T, Tanaka T (1996) Light and electron microscopic studies of bone-titanium interface in the tibiae of young and mature rats. J Biomed Mater Res 30:523–533

50. Meyer U, Joos U, Mythili J, Stamn T, Hohoff A, Fillies T, Stratmann U, Wiesman HP (2004) Ultrastructural characterization of the implant/bone interface of immediately loaded dental implants. Biomaterials 25:1959–1967

51. Puleo DA, Nanci A (1999) Understanding and controlling the bone implant interface. Biomaterials 20:2311–2321

52. Shen X, Roberts E, Peel SAF, Davies JE (1993) Organic extracellular matrix components at the bone cell/substratum interface. Cell Mater 3:257–272

53. Peel SAF (1995) The influence of substratum modification on interfacial bone formation in vitro. Ph.D. Thesis, University of Toronto

54. Gorsky JP (1998) Is all bone the same? Distinctive distributions and properties of non-collagenous matrix proteins in lamellar vs. woven bone imply the existence of different underlying osteogenic mechanisms. Crit Rev Oral Biol Med 9:201–223

55. Davies JE (2003) Understanding peri-implant endosseous healing. J Dent Educ 67:932–949

56. Rosengren A, Johanson BR, Danielsen N, Thomsen P, Ericson LE (1996) Immunohistochemical studies on the distribution of albumin, fibrinogen, fibronectin, IgG and collagen around PTFE and titanium implants. Biomaterials 17:1779–1786

57. Pritchard JJ (1972) General histology of bone. In: Bourne GH (ed) The biochemistry and physiology of bone, vol 120. Academic, New York
58. Parfitt AM (1983) The physiology and clinical significance of bone histomorphometric data. In: Recker RR (ed) Bone histomorphometry: techniques and interpretation. CRC, Boca Raton, pp 143–223
59. Villanueva AR, Sypitkowski C, Parfitt AM (1986) A new method for identification of cement lines in undecalcified, plastic embedded sections of bone. Stain Technol 61:83–88
60. Frasca P (1981) Scanning electron microscopy study of ground substance in the cement lines, resting lines, hypercalcified rings and reversal lines of human cortical bone. Acta Anat 109:115–121
61. McKee MD, Nanci A (1993) Ultrastrucutural, Cytochemical and immunocytochemical studies on bone and its interface. Cell Mater 3:219–243
62. Butler WT (1989) The nature and significance of osteopontin. Connect Tissue Res 23:123–136
63. Linder L (1985) High-resolution microscopy of the implant-tissue interface. Acta Orthop Scand 56:269–272
64. Albrektsson T, Hansson HA (1986) An ultrastructural characterization of the interface between bone and sputtered titanium or stainless steel surfaces. Biomaterials 7:201–205
65. Davies J, Lowenberg B, Shiga A (1990) The bone-titanium interface in vitro. J Biomed Mater Res 24:1289–1306
66. Probst A, Spiegel HU (1997) Cellular mechanisms of bone repair. J Invest Surg 10:77–86
67. Roberts WE (1988) Bone tissue interface. J Dent Educ 52:804–809
68. Linder L, Obrant K, Boivin G (1989) Osseointegration of metallic implants II. Transmission electron microscopy in the rabbit. Acta Orthop Scand 60:135–139
69. Clokie CML, Warshawsky H (1995) Morphologic and radioautographic studies of bone formation in relation to titanium implants using rat tibia as a model. Int J Oral Maxillofac Implants 10:155–165
70. Davies JE, Hosseini MM (2000) Histodynamics of endosseous wound healing. In: Davies JE (ed) Bone engineering. Em Squared Inc, Toronto, pp 1–14
71. Davies JE, Chernecky R, Lowenberg B, Shiga A (1991) Deposition and resorption of calcified matrix in vitro by rat bone marrow cells. Cells Mater 1:3–15
72. von Ebner (Ritter von Rosenheim) V (1875) Über den feineren Bau der Knochensubstanz (On the fine structure of bone) SB Akad Wiss Math Kl Abt III 72:49–138
73. Morinaga K, Kido H, Sato A, Watazu A, Matsuura M (2009) Chronological changes in the ultrastructure of titanium-bone interfaces: analysis by light microscopy, transmission electron microscopy, and micro-computed tomography. Clin Implant Dent Relat Res 11:59–68
74. Schwartz Z, Lohmann CH, Vocke AK, Sylvia VL, Cochran DL, Dean DD, Boyan BD (2001) Osteoblast response to titanium surface roughness and 1alpha,25-(OH)(2)D(3) is mediated through the mitogen-activated protein kinase (MAPK) pathway. J Biomed Mater Res 56:417–426
75. Orsini G, Assenza B, Scarano A, Piattelli M, Piattelli A (2000) Surface analysis of machined versus sandblasted and acid-etched titanium implants. Int J Oral Maxillofac Implants 15:779–784
76. Boyan BD, Bonewald LF, Paschalis EP, Lohmann CH, Rosser J, Cochran DL, Dean DD, Schwartz Z, Boskey AL (2002) Osteoblastmediated mineral deposition in culture is dependent on surface microtopography. Calcif Tissue Int 71:519–529
77. Lohmann CH, Sagun R Jr, Sylvia VL, Cochran DL, Dean DD, Boyan BD, Schwartz Z (1999) Surface roughness modulates the response of MG63 osteoblast-like cells to 1,25-(OH)(2)D(3) through regulation of phospholipase A(2) activity and activation of protein kinase A. J Biomed Mater Res 47:139–151
78. Park JY, Gemmell CH, Davies JE (2001) Platelets interactions with titanium: modulation of platelet activity by surface topography. Biomaterials 22:2671–2682
79. Soskolne WA, Cohen S, Sennerby L, Wennebrg A, Shapira L (2002) The effect of titanium surface roughness on the adhesion of monocytes and their secretion of TNF-a and PGE 2. Clin Oral Implants Res 13:86–93

80. Albrektsson T, Wennerberg A (2004) Oral implant surfaces: Part 2- review focusing on clinical knowledge of different surfaces. Int J Prosthodont 17:544–564
81. Zechner W, Tangl S, Furst G, Tepper G, Thams U, Mailath G, Watzek G (2003) Ossoeus healing characteristics of three different implant types. Clin Oral Implants Res 14:150–157
82. Cook SD, Thomas KA, Kay JF, Jarcho M (1988) Hydroxyapatite coated porous titanium for use as an orthopaedic biologic attachment system. Clin Orthop 230:303–312
83. Shirakura M, Fujii N, Ohnishi H, Taguchi Y, Ohshima H, Nomura S, Maeda T (2003) Tissue response to titanium implantation in the rat maxilla, with special reference to the effect of surface conditions on bone formation. Clin Oral Implant Res 14:687–696
84. Ducheyne P, Healy KE (1988) The effect of plasma sprayed calcium phosphate ceramic coatings on the metal ion release from titanium and cobalt chromium alloys. J Biomed Mater Res 22:1137–1163
85. Martini D, Fini M, Franchi M, De Pasquale V, Bacchelli B, Gamberoni M, Tinti A, Taddei P, Giavaresi G, Ottani V, Raspanti M, Guizzard S, Ruggeri A (2003) Detachment of titanium and fluorohydroxyapatite particles in unloaded endosseous implants. Biomaterials 4:1309–1316
86. Jones FH (2001) Teeth and bones: applications of surface science to dental materials and related biomaterials. Surf Sci Rep 42:75–205
87. Wheeler SL (1996) Eight-year clinical retrospective study of titanium plasma-sprayed and hydroxyapatite-coated cylinder implants. Int J Oral Maxillofac Implants 11:340–350
88. Geesink RG, de Groot K, Klein CP (1988) Bonding of bone to apatite coated implants. J Bone Joint Surg Br 70:17–22
89. Chang YL, Lew D, Park JB, Keller J (1999) Biomechanical and morphometric analysis of hydroxyapatite-coated implants with varying crystallinity. J Oral Maxillofac Surg 57:1096–1108
90. Galoi L, Mainard D (2004) Bone ingrowth into two porous ceramics with different pore sizes: an experimental study. Acta Orthop Belg 70:598–603
91. Park YS, Yi KY, Lee IS, Han CH, Jumg YC (2005) The effects of ion beam-assisted deposition of hydroxyapatite on the grit-blasted surface of endosseous implants in rabbit tibiae. Int J Oral Maxillofac Implants 20:31–38
92. Vercaigne S, Wolke JGC, Naert I, Jansen JA (1998) The effect of titanium plasma-sprayed implants on trabecular bone healing in the goat. Biomaterials 19:1093–1099
93. Hansson S (1999) The implant neck: smooth or provided with retention elements. A biomechanical approach. Clin Oral Implants Res 10:394–405

Author Index

A
Abad, V., 23
Abate, C., 21
Abboud, H.E., 61
Abboud, S.L., 88
Abboud-Werner, S., 61
Abou-Samra, A.B., 27
Abrahamsson, I., 120
Abu-Lafi, S., 69
Adams, C.S., 120
Adams, S.L., 25
Adell, R., 119
Afzal, F., 20
Agapitos, E., 56
Agrogiannis, G., 56
Aguiar, D.J., 12
Ahdjoudj, S., 12
Ahn, J.D., 21
Ahrlund-Richter, L., 86
Ai-Aql, Z.S., 5
Ailhaud, G., 86
Aizawa, T., 3
Akagawa, Y., 103
Akao, Y., 23
Akbas, F., 68
Akira, S., 19
Akiyama, H., 19
Alagl, A.S., 5
Albig, W., 53
Alblas, J., 104, 105, 107
Alblowi, J., 61, 62
Albrektsson, T., 119, 121, 122
Albright, S., 16, 17
Aldahmash, A., 87
Alexander, J.M., 52
Alexandrovich, A., 69
Ali, A.A., 18, 19

Ali, S.Y., 43
Allen, B., 61
Alman, B.A., 6
Almeida, M., 61
Al-Sebaei, M.O., 61
Al-Zube, L., 61
Amanat, N., 32
Ambrosetti, D., 22
Amedee, J., 120
Amemiya, T., 23
Amir, D., 44
Amir, G., 59–63
Amling, M., 21
Amor, S., 72, 73
Amsel, S., 52
Anastopoulos, G., 56
Andersen, T.L., 30
Anderson, D.M., 29
Anderson, H.C., 43
Ando, F., 75
Andrade, A.C., 26
Andreassen, T.T., 52, 100
Andriamanalijaona, R., 91
An, D.S., 89
Angel, P., 19
Aoki, K., 21
Aoyama, I., 100, 106, 107
Aponte-Wesson, R., 63
Apparailly, F., 11
Appleford, M., 120
Arai, F., 29
Arana-Chavez, V.E., 63
Armitage, J.E., 119
Arnaud, C., 68
Arnaud, E., 100, 105
Arnol, V., 63
Aro, H.T., 101

J.J. Sela and I.A. Bab (eds.), *Principles of Bone Regeneration*,
DOI 10.1007/978-1-4614-2059-0, © Springer Science+Business Media, LLC 2012

Aronin, N., 21
Aronow, M., 16
Arriagada, G., 18
Arron, J.R., 28
Asagiri, M., 19, 20, 28
Asahina, I., 100
Ashhurst, D.E., 3, 4, 6, 53
Asimakopoulos, A., 56
Aslan, H., 83, 85, 89
Aspenberg, P., 56
Assenza, B., 121
Astrup, A., 68
Atsuta, M., 120
Attar-Namdar, M., 53
Attawia, M.A., 85, 87
Aubert, J.F., 68, 71
Aubin, J.E., 102
Augat, P., 102
Avioli, L.V., 22, 83, 102
Ayer, D.E., 21
Aylsworth, A.S., 16, 17
Ayukawa, Y., 120, 121
Azad, V., 62
Azar, P., 63
Azzarà, A., 53
Azzar, G., 44

B
Bab, I.A., 1–7, 11–32, 43, 44,
    51–56, 67–75
Bacchelli, B., 120, 122
Badihi, L., 120
Bae, I.H., 18
Bae, J.S., 20
Bae, S.C., 18, 20
Bae, Y.C., 18
Bahamonde, M.E., 83, 87, 89
Bai, J., 61
Bailey, J., 18, 19
Bailly, S., 86
Bain, G., 22
Bain, S.D., 87
Bai, X.C., 61
Baker, D., 68, 72, 73
Balanika, A., 56
Balcerzak, M., 43, 44
Balian, G., 60
Ballester, A.H., 63
Ballock, T.R., 23, 26, 27
Bandorowicz-Pikula, J., 44
Banerjee, C., 21
Banfi, A., 111
Bank, R.A., 86

Banks, B.A., 120
Barbosa, A.C., 18
Barlogie, B., 22
Barnes, G.L., 3, 52
Barnes, K.M., 23
Baron, J., 23, 25, 26
Baron, R., 21, 22
Barrilleaux, B., 102
Barrio, D.A., 63
Bar-Shavit, Z., 28
Barth, F., 68
Basilico, C., 22
Batista, A.C., 62
Bátkai, S., 69
Battle, M.A., 104, 106
Bauer, M.A., 61
Baumann, B., 19
Bay, B.H., 104
Baylink, D.J., 99
Beam, H.A., 60–62
Beastall, G., 56
Bechkoff, G., 44
Becker, M., 19
Beck, S.C., 82
Beddington, R.S., 16, 17
Behrens, J., 21
Behringer, R.R., 15, 16, 19
Beirne, O.R., 104
Bellahcene, A., 18
Bellantuono, I., 87
Bellido, T., 18, 19
Bellini, G., 69
Bellows, C.G., 102
Bell, R., 104
Belmonte, N., 86
Benabdallah, B.F., 91
Benayahu, D., 102
Benit, P., 20
Bennett, L., 29
Ben-Shabat, S., 68, 69
Berend, M.E., 62
Beresford, J.N., 102
Berger, R., 26
Bergin, I., 98, 107
Berglundh, T., 120
Bertoncello, I., 32
Beslot, F., 68, 71
Bessho, K., 100, 120
Betz, O., 7
Bhat, R.A., 22
Bialek, P., 19–21
Bianchi, G., 111
Bianco, P., 91, 98, 99, 102, 110
Bigey, P., 91

Bikle, D.D., 27
Billin, A.N., 21
Binon, P., 119
Birchmeier, W., 21
Birnbaum, M.J., 53
Bishop, G.B., 83
Bisogno, T., 68, 69
Bi, W., 15, 16
Blackstad, M., 86
Bland, Y.S., 3, 4
Blavier, L., 30
Bloch-Zupan, A., 20
Blotter, R.H., 60
Blumenfeld, I., 102, 106
Blum, W., 26
Bode, C., 53
Boden, S.D., 83, 91
Bodine, P.V., 22
Boering, G., 23
Boheler, K.R., 86
Bohner, M., 104
Boivin, G., 121
Bokko, P., 60
Bolander, M.E., 60
Bolcato-Bellemin, A.L., 20
Bolognesi, M.P., 62
Boman, A., 26
Bonaventure, J., 20
Bond, A.T., 27
Bonewald, L.F., 100, 121
Bonner, T.I., 75
Bonucci, E., 43
Boone, T., 29
Bortell, R., 21
Bosch, C., 7, 106
Bosch, P., 82, 85, 87, 89
Boskey, A.L., 121
Botchwey, E.A., 106
Botolin, S., 61
Bouaboula, M., 68
Bouali, Y., 21
Bouchard, L.S., 107
Bouchentouf, M., 91
Boules, H., 19
Boumah, C.E., 19
Bourgeois, P., 20
Bowen, C.V., 23
Boyan, B.D., 25, 44, 120–122
Boyer, M.I., 23
Boyle, W.J., 29, 30
Brabbs, A., 30
Bracey, M.H., 69
Bradica, G., 61
Braidman, I.P., 87

Brancorsini, S., 19
Branemark, P.I., 119
Breine, U., 119
Breitbart, E.A., 61
Breuer, A., 68, 69
Bridgen, D.T., 69
Bringhurst, F.R., 25
Brondello, J.M., 11
Bronson, R.T., 16, 17
Brown, J.P., 75
Brown, M.K., 105
Bruce, A.G., 106, 107
Bruce, W., 105
Bruder, S.P., 4, 85, 107
Bruhn, L., 21
Bruzzone, L., 63
Bucay, N., 29
Buchet, R., 43, 44
Buckwalter, J.A., 82
Buhner, M., 120
Bunger, C., 99, 100, 104, 106
Bunn, R.C., 60
Burger, E.H., 100
Burger, F., 68
Burgess, T., 30
Burridge, K., 120
Butler, W.T., 121
Byers, R.J., 87
Byrne, M., 53

C
Cadide, T., 75
Calandra, B., 68
Calmar, E.A., 23
Cameron, H.U., 120
Caminis, J., 75
Campbell, P., 29
Canalis, E., 101
Cancedda, R., 98, 111
Cao, Y., 56
Caplan, A.I., 1, 5, 83, 105
Capparelli, C., 30
Carillo, F., 75
Carlson, A.E., 22
Carmines, D., 60
Carpi, A., 120
Carrascal, M.T., 56
Carter, D.R., 120
Caruso, E.M., 1, 5
Caruso, T., 102, 108
Casap, N., 53, 63
Cascino, J.E., 18
Cascio, M.G., 69

Casellas, P., 68
Castilla, L.H., 86
Castronovo, V., 18
Cathepsin, K., 32
Cavalher-Machado, S.C., 63
Cecchini, M.G., 21
Cecil, R.N.A., 43
Celeste, A.J., 53, 83, 100
Centrella, M., 101
Cerami, A., 63
César-Neto, J.B., 75
Cha, B.S., 62
Chaffin, D.G., 25
Chailakhyan, R.K., 52
Chai, Y., 21
Cha, J.M., 108
Chambers, T.J., 61
Champagne, N., 18
Chang, H.C., 61
Chang, J., 21
Chang, M.S., 29
Chang, W., 27
Chang, Y.L., 122
Chan, K.L., 108
Chapman, M.W., 60
Chapman-Sheath, P., 105
Chapuy, M.C., 75
Chaudhari, A., 83
Chaudhary, S.B., 62
Chavali, R., 63
Chen, D., 18, 20
Chen, G., 21
Cheng, S.L., 22, 83, 102
Chen, H.Y., 68
Chen, J.T., 7, 21, 61
Chen, L.F., 20
Chen, M., 20
Chen, R.M., 61
Chen, S.T., 89
Chen, T.F., 61
Chen, T.L., 61
Chen, Y.C., 6, 53, 83
Chernecky, R., 121
Cheung, K.M., 83
Chiang, L.C., 20
Chissas, D., 56
Chiusaroli, R., 21
Chi, X.Z., 20
Cho, H.H., 18
Choi, H.R., 18
Choi, H.S., 18
Choi, J.Y., 16–18, 20, 85, 86
Choi, N.S., 18
Choi, Y., 28

Cho, K., 19
Chong, E.J., 104
Choo, M.K., 18, 20
Chorev, M., 12, 15, 52–54
Cho, T.J., 3
Choy, L., 85, 86
Chrysis, D., 26
Chua, S.C., 19
Chung, U.I., 25
Cimino, C.D., 120
Cimino, G., 102, 108
Claes, L., 102
Clark, R.M., 25
Clevers, H., 21
Clokie, C.M.L., 120, 121
Cnudde, V., 103, 105, 108
Cochran, D.L., 120–122
Cogan, J., 21
Cohen, A.J., 25
Cohen, S., 122
Cohen-Solal, M., 75
Cole, W.G., 16, 17
Collart, D., 16
Collyer, J., 100
Colombero, A., 29, 30
Colvin, J.S., 26
Composto, R.J., 120
Conlon, D., 102
Conner, D.A., 25, 26
Connolly, E., 60
Conte, A., 53
Cook, C., 60
Cook, S.D., 120, 122
Cooper, G.M., 85
Cornelissen, M., 107
Cornell, C.N., 98, 104
Correa, D., 22
Corsari, V., 120
Cortizo, A.M., 63
Cory, E., 7
Cossu, G., 68, 71
Costantini, F., 26
Coulier, F., 26
Courey, A.J., 21
Cravatt, B.F., 69
Criswell, B., 21
Critchlow, M.A., 3, 4
Croce, C.M., 23
Crompton, T., 16, 17
Cronin, M.T., 61
Crosby, W.H., 52
Crossan, J.F., 56
Cruzat, F., 18
Csimma, C., 83

Culbertson, K.C., 120
Cunningham, M., 91
Cutler, G.B., 26

D
D'Alessandro, J.S., 83
Dallas, J.S., 25, 27
D'Alonzo, R.C., 19
Daluiski, A., 83, 87, 89
Damsky, C.H., 120, 121
D'Angelo, A.M., 120
Dani, C., 86
Daniels, D.L., 21
Danielsen, N., 121
Danse, J.M., 20
da Silva, T.A., 62
Davey, M.R., 91
David, J.P., 21
David, L., 86
Davies, J., 121
Davies, J.E., 98, 106, 120–122
Davies, J.T., 61
Davis, J.B., 68
Davy, E., 29, 30
Dayoub, H., 83
Deakin, M., 105
de Amorim, F.P., 62
Dean, D.D., 25, 121, 122
Dean, J.W. 3rd., 120
Deasy, B.M., 82, 85
Debes, J., 105
De Bont, L.G.M., 23
Debouck, C., 32
de Crombrugghe, B., 15, 16, 19, 20
Deeds, J.D., 27
de Groot, K., 122
Deguchi, K., 16, 17
Delaisse, J.M., 30
Delaney, J., 30
Delany, A.M., 23
De Levi, S., 23
Delgado, C.G., 20
Delgado-Martinez, A.D., 56
Deligianni, D.D., 120
Delmas, P.D., 75
De Luca, F., 23, 25
de Luna, R.I.O., 20
Demarest, K., 69
Demer, L.L., 18
de Morais, J.A., 63
Deng, J.M., 19
Dennis, J.E., 83
Dennison, D., 120

Denzel, A., 16, 17
de Oliveira, P.T., 120
De Paepe, I., 103
De Pasquale, V., 120, 122
De Petrocellis, L., 68, 69
Derby, P., 29
DeRose, M., 29
Derynck, R., 85, 86
Destree, O., 21
Detry, C., 18
De Ugarte, D.A., 85, 86
Deutsch, D., 43, 44
Devados, R., 20
Devane, W.A., 68
Devlin, V.J., 52, 53
Devoto, M., 75
de Wijn, J.R., 104, 105
Dhert, W.J., 104, 105, 107
Dijkgraaf, L.C., 23
Di Marzo, V., 68, 69
Dimitriou, R., 3
Diniz, S.F., 62
D'Ippolito, G., 98, 102, 108
Dixon, A., 21
Djouad, F., 11
Dobner, P.R., 21
Dodds, R., 32
Doenecke, D., 53
Doi, K., 103
Domene, H.M., 26
Dong, Y., 19
Donley, B.G., 62
Doty, S.B., 27, 120, 121
Doulabi, B.Z., 86
Doumas, C., 61
Drabent, B., 53
Dragoo, J.L., 85, 86
Drake, F., 32
Drissi, H., 19
Dubruel, P., 103, 105,
        107, 108
Ducheyne, P., 105, 120, 122
Duguy, N., 100, 105
Dulai, S., 32
Dumont, R.J., 83
Dunn, F., 22
Dunstan, C.R., 29, 30
Duroux-Richard, I., 11

E
Ebara, S., 83
Ebner, R., 87
Edouard, C., 75

Edwards, J.R., 56
Efraty, M., 102
Einhorn, T.A., 3–6, 52, 53, 59, 61, 62, 83
Ejersted, C., 52
Elalieh, H.Z., 27
Elbarbary, A., 85, 86
el Ghouzzi, V., 20
Eli, A., 30
Elisseeff, J., 107
Elliott, C., 21
Elliott, G., 30
Elliott, R., 29, 30
Ellis, E.F., 69
Endo, N., 53
Engsig, M.T., 30
Engstrand, T., 83, 87, 89
Ennever, J., 43
Enomoto-Iwamoto, M., 26
Ericson, L.E., 121
Erson, A.E., 23
Esposito, M., 119
Etcheverry, S.B., 63
Ettinger, M.P., 102, 107
Eulenberger, J., 119
Evans, L., 43

F
Fajardo, R., 7
Fang, T.D., 91
Fan, Z., 21
Farinas, I., 21
Faris, P.M., 62
Fazzi, R., 53
Fedorovich, N.E., 104, 105, 107
Fehse, B., 89
Feige, J.J., 86
Feldman, D., 63
Feldman, S.A., 119
Felice, J.I., 63
Felix, R., 21
Feng, X., 22
Fernandez, J., 21
Ferrara, N., 86
Ferreira, E., 91
Ferron, M., 19
Fialkov, J.A., 98, 106
Field, J., 32
Fillies, T., 120
Finazzi-Agro, A., 68
Fini, M., 120, 122
Fink, D.J., 4
Fiorellini, J.P., 63
Fish, S., 52

Flanders, K.C., 101
Fledelius, C., 52
Fleisch, H.A., 21
Fleischman, A.J., 120
Fleming, J.E. Jr., 98, 104
Flores, A., 56
Fogel, M., 69, 72, 73
Follak, N., 60
Fontana, A., 102, 108
Ford, K., 21
Forman, L.J., 100
Fourmousis, I., 63
Fowler, B., 85
Fowler, C.J., 68
Fowlkes, J.L., 60
Franceschi, R.T., 18, 19, 21, 22, 106, 120
Franchi, M., 120, 122
Franke, K., 53
Franke, S., 63
Franz, D.A., 107
Frasca, P., 121
Freed, L.E., 98, 107
Frenkel, B., 21, 53, 69, 72, 73
Freudenberg, J., 75
Fride, E., 68–70
Fried, A., 102
Friedenstein, A.J., 98, 103
Froesch, E.R., 25, 26
Fromigué, O., 12, 83
Fujii, H., 61
Fujii, N., 120, 122
Fujimura, K., 100
Fujioka, H., 60
Fukagawa, M., 61
Fukuda, T., 23
Fuller, K., 61
Funk, J.R., 60
Fu, Q., 18, 19
Furst, G., 122
Furukawa, T., 105
Futami, T., 120

G
Gabarin, N., 53
Gabet, Y., 12, 15, 21, 54, 68, 70
Gafni, R.I., 23
Galimberti, S., 53
Galindo, M., 22
Galoi, L., 122
Galson, D.L., 19
Gamberoni, M., 122
Gamie, Z., 56
Gander, B., 104

Gandhi, A., 60–62
Gangoiti, M.V., 63
Gao, N., 19
Gao, Y.H., 16, 17
Garcia, A.J., 120
Garcia, C.F., 63
Garcia, M., 82, 85
Garimella, R., 43
Garino, J., 105
Garrett, I.R., 56
Gasteyger, C., 68
Gaur, T., 22
Gavenis, K., 53
Gavish, H., 53
Gazit, D., 52, 53, 81–92
Ge, C., 19
Geesink, R.G., 122
Geis-Gerstorfer, J., 120
Gemmell, C.H., 122
Genina, O., 107
Gensac, M.C., 53
George, K.L., 69, 72
Gerasimov, Y.V., 52
Gerber, H.P., 86
Gerstenfeld, L., 61, 62
Gerstenfeld, L.C., 3, 5, 16, 52, 61, 62, 120
Gerstenfeld, L.G., 16
Ghosh-Choudhury, N., 88
Giang, D.K., 69
Giannoudis, P., 3
Giardino, R., 120
Giavaresi, G., 120, 122
Gibbons, R., 106
Gibson, G., 27
Gillespy, T. 3rd., 107
Gillies, R.M., 105
Gilmour, K.C., 16, 17
Giori, N.J., 120
Glass, D.A. 2nd., 21
Glimcher, L.H., 18
Glimcher, M.J., 18
Globus, R.K., 120, 121
Glover, R., 120
Goater, J.J., 88
Godfrey, C., 32
Goldenberg, D., 68
Gombotz, W.R., 107
Gomez, G.T., 75
Gonshor, A., 119
Gonzalez-Ramos, M., 20
Gooch, H.L., 60
Goodman, M., 53
Goodman, S.A., 100
Gopalakrishnan, R., 12, 15, 18, 19, 22

Goparaju, S.K., 69
Gordeladze, J.O., 11
Gori, F., 83
Gorin, Y., 61
Gorsky, J.P., 121
Goto, K., 61, 98
Gowen, M., 32
Graff, J.M., 19
Graham, S., 56
Graves, D.T., 3, 5, 25, 61, 62
Gray, J.C., 43
Greenberg, Z., 52, 53
Green, E.D., 20
Greene, G.W., 119
Greenfield, E.M., 29
Greig, I.R., 68
Grenard, P., 68
Gresnigt, M.G., 26
Griffin, A., 107
Griffin, G., 68
Griffith, C.K., 91
Grigoriadis, A.E., 21
Grodzinsky, A., 98, 107
Groeneveld, E.H., 100
Gronowicz, G., 52
Gronthos, S., 91, 98, 110
Grosschedl, R., 21
Gruber, M., 25, 26
Guan, K., 21
Gubrij, I., 18, 19
Guizzard, S., 122
Guo, J., 25, 30
Guo, W.H., 20
Gutierrez, G.E., 56
Gutierrez, S., 18, 20
Gysin, R., 83

H
Hadi, T., 100
Hale, J.E., 60
Hallen, J., 119
Halloran, B.P., 27
Hamada, Y., 61
Hamade, E., 44
Hamers, N., 26
Hanada, K., 83, 100
Hanai, J., 20
Hanauer, A., 19
Han, C.D., 62
Han, C.H., 122
Hansson, B.O., 119
Hansson, H.-A., 119, 121
Hansson, S., 122

Hanus, A.L., 68
Hanus, L., 68, 69
Harada, T., 20
Harris, B.H., 60
Harrison, J., 105
Harrison, R.J., 21
Hart, B., 72, 73
Hart, C.E., 61
Hartmann, C., 25, 26
Hasegawa, H., 63
Hasegawa, S., 98, 105
Hasharoni, A., 83, 90
Hashimoto, K., 63
Hashimoto, N., 105–107
Hassan, M.Q., 22, 23
Hauschka, P.V., 100
Hawkins, N., 30
Hawse, J.R., 22
Hayashi, K., 103
Hayashi, M., 19, 20
Hayes, W.C., 85, 104, 106, 107, 119
Healy, K.E., 122
Hebb, A.L., 75
Heberer, M., 98, 107
Hecht, A., 21
Heersche, J.N., 102
Hegde, A., 26
Heijink, A., 86
Hein, G., 63
Heino, T.J., 30
Heinrichs, C., 26
Heinze, E., 25
Helder, M.N., 86
Helebrant, A., 120
Helm, G.A., 83, 90
Helms, J.A., 1, 2, 5
Hennink, W.E., 105, 107
Henn, W., 16, 17
Henriksen, K., 30
Henrotin, Y., 18
Hentunen, T.A., 30
Herbertson, A., 102
Herbsman, H., 60, 61
Herkenham, M., 75
Hertzog, P., 32
Hesse, E., 22
Hess, J., 75
Hewick, R.M., 100
Hicok, K.C., 83
Higgins, T., 19
Higuchi, T., 104, 107
Hilbe, M., 7
Hile, D.D., 106

Hill, D., 29
Hille, B., 68
Hillebrands, J.L., 63
Hill, T.P., 25, 26
Hinoi, E., 19
Hirata, K., 120
Hirsch, J.-M., 119
Hirschman, A., 60, 61
Hishikawa, Y., 120
Ho, A.M., 85
Hocker, H., 120
Hoeppner, L.H., 22
Hofmann, S., 7, 83
Hofstaetter, J.G., 18
Hofstetter, W., 21
Hogan, P.G., 20
Hohmann, A.G., 68, 75
Hohoff, A., 120
Hollinger, J.O., 102, 109
Holmes, G., 22
Holmuhamedov, E., 120, 121
Holst, M., 26
Holt, G., 56
Holy, C.E., 98, 106
Holzman, L., 52, 53
Hong, J.J., 61
Hong, L., 105–107
Hong, N., 20
Horn, D., 61
Horne, W.C., 22
Horowitz, M.C., 7, 68
Hoshi, K., 25
Hosseini, M.M., 121
Hou, S.C., 26
Hovhannisyan, H., 22
Howard, G.A., 98
Howard, T.D., 20
Howell, F., 69
Howlett, A.C., 68, 72, 73
Hoyland, J.A., 87
Hsu, H.H.T., 30, 43
Hsu, W.K., 86
Huang, W., 15, 16
Huang, Y., 19
Huard, J., 82, 85, 87, 89
Hugel, U., 26
Hughes, F.J., 100
Hughes, T.M., 29
Hu, H., 75
Hulth, A., 100
Humphries, M.J., 120, 121
Hurwitz, S.A., 60
Hurwitz, S.R., 60

Hutmacher, D.W., 107
Hwang, Y.S., 108
Hynes, R.O., 99

I
Ichinohe, N., 100
Idris, A.I., 68, 69
Idusuyi, O.B., 62
Iglesias, R., 85, 86
Iizuka, T., 100
Ikada, Y., 105–107
Ikeda, T., 120
Imamura, T., 19, 20
Impivaara, O., 60
Imschenetzky, M., 18
Inada, M., 16, 17
Ishidou, Y., 20
Ishiguro, H., 75
Ishii, S., 105
Ishikawa, I., 104, 107
Ishizuya, T., 83
Itoh, T., 23
Ito, K., 20
Ito, Y., 20
Iversen, L., 68
Iwamoto, K., 29
Iwamoto, M., 26
Iwata, K., 56

J
Jabs, E.W., 20
Jacobs, P.J., 103, 105, 108
Jacquot, S., 19
Jagger, C.J., 61
Jahagirdar, B.N., 82, 86
Jaiswal, N., 85, 107
Jankowski, R.J., 82, 85
Jansen, J.A., 100, 119, 122
Járai, Z., 69
Jarcho, M., 122
Javed, A., 16–18, 20, 22
Jayaraman, M., 120
Jefcoat, S.C., 19
Jensen, E.D., 12, 15–19, 22
Jensen, J.B., 68
Jeon, E.J., 18
Jeong, B.C., 18
Jiang, D., 19
Jiang, Y., 19, 82, 86, 100
Jilka, R.L., 18, 19
Jimbo, R., 120

Jingushi, S., 60
Jin, T., 61
Jin, Y.H., 18
Jochum, W., 21
Johanson, B.R., 121
Jones, D.C., 18
Jones, F.H., 122
Joos, U., 120
Jorgensen, C., 11
Jr, C., 23, 26
Julien, B., 68
Jumg, Y.C., 122
Jundt, G., 98, 107
Jung, D.Y., 19
Jung, J.S., 18
Juppner, H., 27
Justice, M.J., 20
Jux, C., 26

K
Kacena, M.A., 7
Kadiyala, S., 85, 107
Kadowaki, T., 25
Kaestner, K.H., 19
Kagami, H., 108
Kagel, E.M., 59
Kahler, R.A., 18, 21, 22
Kahn, A., 87
Kajimura, D., 19
Kaji, Y., 56
Kakar, S., 52, 61
Kalajzic, I., 89
Kalajzic, Z., 89
Kaminski, N.E., 68
Kana, S.M., 60
Kanatani, N., 26
Kaneda, Y., 20
Kaneki, H., 20
Kanesaki, Y.Y., 23
Kanno, T., 20
Kapadia, R., 32
Kapinas, K., 23
Kaplan, D.L., 7
Karageorgiou, V., 83
Karimbux, N.Y., 63
Karmish, M., 52, 53
Karner, E., 86
Karoussis, I.K., 63
Karsak, M., 68, 69, 72, 73, 75
Karsenty, G., 18–21, 25
Kasemo, B., 120, 121
Kashiwagi, K., 20

Kassem, M., 87
Katayama, R., 88
Kato, H., 20
Kato, M., 86
Kato, R., 26
Katsala, N., 120
Kaufman, D.S., 82
Kaufman, S., 30
Kawabata, M., 20
Kawaguchi, H., 25, 100
Kayal, R.A., 61, 62
Kay, J.F., 122
Kazakos, K., 56
Kazarian, S.G., 108
Keating, M.E., 62
Keenan, B.S., 25, 27
Keller, J., 100, 122
Kelley, M.J., 29, 30
Kelley, P., 82–84, 87
Kelly, M.E., 75
Kelz, M.B., 21
Kemler, R., 21
Kempen, D.H., 86
Kemp, S.F., 60
Kenmotsu, S., 25
Kern, B., 20
Kern, D., 120
Kern, T., 120
Kessler, C.B., 23
Kesters, M.A., 120
Ke, Z.Y., 61
Khan, A.J., 52
Khan, Y., 98
Khoshhal, K.I., 61
Kibblewhite, D.J., 107
Kido, H., 121
Kikuchi, H., 106, 107
Kim, A.Y., 18
Kim, C.H., 61
Kim, D.K., 18
Kim, D.M., 63
Kim, E.G., 20
Kimelman-Bleich, N., 81–92
Kim, H.J., 20
Kim, H.N., 18
Kim, J.B., 18
Kim, J.K., 19
Kim, K.W., 61
Kim, S.H., 18
Kimura, T., 88
Kim, W.Y., 20
Kim, Y.J., 18
Kindmark, H., 120

Kingman, A., 85
Kinoshita, A., 104, 107
Kintou, N., 83
Kirker-Head, C., 7, 83
Kirkpatrick, C.J., 103, 105, 107, 108
Kirstein, B., 61
Kishimoto, T., 16, 17
Kitagaki, J., 26
Kita, M., 98
Kitamura, M., 105
Kitamura, Y., 16, 17
Kitazawa, R., 61
Kitazawa, S., 61
Kiviranta, R., 22
Kiyoshima, T., 120, 121
Kizhner, T., 98, 106, 108
Klaus, G., 26
Klay, A., 62
Klee, D., 120
Klein, C.P., 122
Klein-Nulend, J., 86
Kleinschmidt, J.C., 109
Kline, A.D., 20
Kline, A.J., 60
Klöting, I., 60
Klöting, L., 60
Knippenberg, M., 86
Knoll, J.H., 16, 17
Knox, I., 25
Kobayashi, T., 25
Kockeritz, L., 21
Kodama, T., 19, 20
Koedam, J.A., 26
Koester, M.C., 56
Kogan, N.M., 68
Koga, T., 19, 20
Kohavi, D., 119–122
Koh, J.T., 18
Kohler, T., 21
Kola, I., 32
Komatsubara, S., 52, 56
Komeda, M., 105, 106
Komiya, S., 19
Komm, B.S., 22
Komori, T., 16, 17, 20, 26
Kondaiah, P., 101
Kondoh, Y., 23
Kon, E., 98
Kon, T., 3
Koo, S.H., 18
Kopman, J.A., 63
Kornak, U., 75
Koster, J.G., 26

Kotsovilis, S., 63
Kowalewski, R., 19
Kowalski, J., 86
Koyama, E., 26
Kozitza, K., 104, 106
Kraus, K.H., 107
Kraut, D., 62
Krebsbach, P.H., 21
Kriz, R.W., 100
Kronenberg, H.M., 25
Krothapalli, N., 61, 62
Kruisbeek, A., 21
Kuboki, Y., 100
Kubo, T., 103
Kuhlcke, K., 89
Kuhl, M., 21
Kundu, R., 21
Kung, H.F., 83
Kung, S.P., 89
Kunkel, G., 19
Kunos, G., 69
Kurokawa, T., 100
Kurth, A.A., 85, 107
Kusakari, H., 120
Kutepov, S.M., 98
Kutner, R., 89
Kuznetsov, S.A., 85, 91, 99, 103
Kveiborg, M., 21
Kwok, S., 19
Kwon, P.T., 63

L
Labat, M.L., 82
L'Abbate, G., 53
Lacey, D.L., 29, 30
Ladas, S., 120
Lagumdzija, A., 120
Lai, C.F., 22
Lai, Y., 19
Lajeunie, E., 20
Lambert, D.M., 68
Lamour, V., 18
Landao-Bassonga, E., 69
Lane, J., 107
Lane, N.E., 100
Langer, B., 119
Langer, R., 7
Lang, N.P., 120
Lang, R.A., 21
Lanske, B., 25
Lanyon, L.E., 30
La Pean, A., 12

Larrabee, W.F. Jr., 106
Larsen, T.M., 68
Lassova, L., 25
Lauckner, J.E., 68
Laurencin, C.T., 85, 87, 98, 106
Lausmaa, J., 120, 121
Lavroukov, A., 98
Lazarus, J.E., 26
Lazner, F., 32
Lazzara, R., 119
Lean, J.M., 61
Leblond, C.P., 103
Lecanda, F., 83
Leclerc, N., 69, 72, 73
Ledent, C., 68, 70, 71
Ledet, T., 100
Lee, C., 21
Lee, H.W., 18, 107
Lee, I.S., 122
Lee, J.M., 61
Lee, J.Y., 85, 87, 89
Lee, K.S., 18, 20, 25, 27
Lee, K.Y., 18
Lee, M.H., 18, 19
Lee, R., 29
Lee, S.C., 104, 106
Lee, S.K., 119
Lee, Y.H., 18
Lee, Y.S., 18
Lefebvre, V., 15, 16
Leiber, K., 26
Leibfritz, D., 61
Leith, J.M., 60
Lekholm, U., 119
Le, L.Q., 83, 87
Lemaitre, J., 104
Le Merrer, M., 20
Lemons, J.E., 63
Lengner, C.J., 22
Lenvik, T., 86
Leo, G., 69
Leone, C.W., 61
Leong, J.C., 83
Lettieri, G., 63
Lettieri, M.G., 63
Le, V., 18
Levine, E.M., 106
Lewandrowski, K.U., 106
Lew, D., 122
Lian, J.B., 16–18, 20–23, 69, 72, 102, 103
Lichtler, A.C., 89
Liebergall, M., 83, 90
Lieberman, J.R., 83, 85–87

Liechty, K.W., 82, 84
Liem, R.S.B., 23
Ligresti, A., 69
Ligumsky, M., 68
Li, J.Z., 83, 91
Li, L., 68
Lilly, L., 83
Lim, C.T., 104
Lim, I.J., 104
Lin, A.C., 6
Linder, L., 121
Linder, T., 56
Lindhe, J., 63, 120
Lindhout, D., 16, 17
Lind, M., 99, 100, 104, 106
Lindsey, W.H., 107
Lindström, J., 119
Lin, G., 82, 85
Links, T., 63
Lin, S.S., 60–62
Lin, Y.L., 61
Liporace, F.A., 62
Lippens, E., 107
Li, Q.L., 19, 20
Listgarten, M.A., 120, 121
Little, D.G., 32, 60
Liu, C., 88
Liu, J., 69
Liu, N.Q., 86
Liu, P., 89
Liu, Y., 91
Liu, Z.J., 82
Livingston, T., 105
Livne, E., 97–111
Li, X.M., 18, 22, 61
Li, Z., 23
Loboa, E.G., 108
Loder, R., 60
Loefler, A., 105
Lohmann, C.H., 120–122
Lombard, C., 27
Lomri, A., 83
London, S.D., 107
Long, F., 21
Losito, I., 106
Lossdorfer, S., 120
Lotz, J., 100
Lou, J., 83, 87
Lou, Y., 20
Lowe, J., 43
Lowe, K.C., 91
Lowenberg, B., 121
Lucas, P.A., 101

Lu, D., 61
Lu, H.C., 62, 68
Luk, K.D., 83
Lu, L., 86
Lull, J.C., 120, 121
Lu, L.Q., 85, 87
Lumpkin, C.K., 60
Luo, M., 19
Luongo, L., 69
Luo, S.Q., 61
Luthy, R., 29
Lu, W.W., 83
Lu, Y., 19
Luzzatto, L., 111
Lyons, J.P., 19
Lyons, K.M., 26, 27, 83, 87, 89

M
MacArthur, C.A., 26
Maccarrone, M., 68
Macey, L.R., 60
Mackay, A.M., 82
MacKenzie, T.C., 82, 84
Mackie, K., 68
Macnab, I., 120
Maeda, S., 19
Maeda, T., 120, 122
Maeusll, P.A., 119
Mailath, G., 122
Mainard, D., 122
Malaval, L., 75
Maloney, M.A., 52
Ma, N., 20
Manabe, T., 56
Maniatis, A., 52
Maniatopoulos, C., 102, 103
Mankani, M.H., 85, 91, 103
Manolagas, S.C., 18, 19, 61
Manske, P., 83, 87
Mansky, K.C., 22
Manson, P.N., 107
Mansukhani, A., 22
Mansur, N., 53
Mantalaris, A., 108
Ma, P.X., 120
Marcacci, M., 98
Marcantonio, E., 63
Marchant, M.H., 62
Margevicius, K., 102
Marie, P.J., 12, 83
Marino, R., 23, 25
Markose, E., 16

Martin, B.R., 69
Martinez, M.E., 56
Martin, I., 98, 107
Martini, D., 120, 122
Martin, J.A., 82
Martin, R.E., 26
Martin, T.J., 99, 105
Marukawa, K., 104
Marx, J., 68
Marzona, L., 1, 2, 5
Mashiba, T., 52, 56
Massarawa, A., 52
Masschaele, B., 103, 107
Mastrogiacomo, M., 98, 111
Masuda, S., 105
Masuoka, H.C., 19
Mata, A., 120
Matsuda, K., 18, 19
Matsui, Y., 19, 20
Matsuno, H., 88
Matsuo, K., 21
Matsusue, Y., 105
Matsuura, M., 121
Mattie, J., 62
Mazur, M., 61
McAnally, J., 18
McCabe, L.R., 21, 61
McCarthy, A.D., 63
McCarthy, G.F., 120
McCarthy, T.L., 101
McCauley, L., 21
McCaw, E., 75
Mccluskey, B., 56
McCool, J., 7
McCormack, R.G., 60
McCracken, M.S., 63
McCrea, P.D., 19
McDonald, M.M., 32, 60
McDougall, K.E., 26
McEwen, D.G., 26
McIntosh, K.R., 103
McKay, R., 103
McKee, M.D., 4, 121
McKe, M.D., 120
McKenzie, E., 61, 62
McKinstry, M.B., 90
Mclellan, A.R., 56
McMahon, A.P., 21, 25
Meadows, E., 18
Mechoulam, R., 68, 69, 72, 73
Meding, J.B., 62
Meenaghan, M.A., 119
Meerwaldt, R., 63

Mehls, O., 26
Meijlink, F., 21
Meinel, L., 7
Meites, J., 100
Melcher, A.H., 102, 103
Melck, D., 69
Melhus, H., 83, 87, 89
Mellado-Valero, A., 63
Melsen, B., 7, 106
Melsen, F., 100
Mercer, N., 63
Merkel, K., 83, 87
Merk, H., 60
Merkle, H.P., 7, 104
Merrell, G.A., 7
Mertelsmann, R., 16, 17
Metelli, M.R., 53
Meunier, P.J., 75
Meyers, J.L., 23
Meyer, U., 120
Meyle, J., 63
Michael, M., 23, 26
Miguel, S.M., 53
Mikos, A.G., 98, 105
Miller, C., 91
Miller, S.K., 120
Minassi, A., 69
Minne, H.W., 52, 53
Mische, S., 21
Missirlis, Y.F., 120
Mitsock, L.M., 100
Miyamoto, K., 56
Miyamoto, S., 105–107
Miyamoto, T., 29
Miyatake, S., 100
Miyazaki, M., 89
Miyazono, K., 20
Mi, Z., 89
Mizrahi, O., 81–92
Mizuno, Y., 23
Mohan, S., 61, 99
Moncol, J., 61
Monsonego-Ornan, E., 107
Montecino, M., 16–18, 22
Moon, H.K., 62
Moon, S.K., 61
Moore, D.C., 83
Moore, S.F., 69
Morgan, E.F., 52, 61
Morieux, C., 75
Morinaga, K., 121
Mori, S., 52, 56
Morizono, K., 85, 86

Morrey, B.F., 62
Morvan, F., 22
Mosca, J.D., 103, 107
Mosley, J.R., 30
Moutsatsos, I.K., 53, 83, 84, 86, 87, 90
Moxham, J.P., 107
Mueller, M., 52, 53
Mueller, R., 52
Muhlrad, A., 43, 44, 52, 53
Mukhachev, V., 98
Mukhopadhyay, K., 21
Mulari, M., 32
Mulhall, D., 43
Müller, R., 12, 15, 21, 54, 68, 70, 84, 85,
    87–89
Muller, T., 22
Mulliken, J.B., 16, 17
Mundlos, C., 16, 17
Mundlos, S., 16, 17
Mundy, G.R., 18, 56, 100
Munnich, A., 20
Munuera, L., 56
Murai, K., 120, 121
Murakami, C.S., 106
Murakami, S., 15, 16
Murray, J., 88
Muruganandan, S., 12, 13
Muschler, G.F., 98, 104
Musgrave, D.S., 82, 85, 87, 89
Myers, M.G. Jr., 19
Mythili, J., 120

N
Nadesan, P., 6
Naert, I., 122
Nagamani, M., 25, 27
Nagarkatti, M., 27
Nagarkatti, P., 27
Nagata, I., 106, 107
Nahounou, M., 52
Nair, A.K., 16, 17
Nakagawa, K., 104
Nakajima, A., 61
Nakajima, F., 61
Nakamura, K., 25, 100
Nakamura, R., 108
Nakamura, T., 19, 98, 105
Nakashima, K., 19, 20
Nakayama, K., 83
Nakazawa, F., 88
Namdar-Attar, M., 53
Namdar, M., 52, 53

Nanci, A., 120, 121
Nardone, J., 20
Narla, R., 20
Natiella, J.R., 119
Nazarian, A., 7
Neff, L., 21, 22
Neidre, D.B., 56
Neiva, T.G., 75
Neo, M., 98, 105
Nestler, E.J., 21
Nevins, M., 119
Nevo, Z ., 54
Ng, K.W., 99
Nguyen, H.Q., 29
Nguyen, T., 99, 104, 106
Nicholson, G.C., 99
Nicolini, A., 120
Nielsen, H.M., 100
Nilsson, O., 23, 25, 26
Nimri, S., 63
Nimura, K., 20
Ning, H., 82, 85
Ninomiya, Y., 23
Nishida, S., 27
Nishimura, I., 100
Nishimura, K., 105, 106
Nishimura, R., 22
Nishino, N., 18
Nishio, Y, 19
Nissenson, R.A., 53
Niyibizi, C., 89
Noble, B.S., 30
Nociti, F.H. Jr., 75
Noël, D., 11
Nogueira-Filho, G.R., 75
Noh, T., 21, 53
Nomura, S., 16, 17, 120, 122
Nooh, N., 3
Notaro, R., 111
Notelovitz, M., 87
Nozawa, Y., 23
Ntagiopoulos, P.G., 56
Nyman, J.S., 56

O
Obrant, K., 121
O'Brien, C.A., 18, 19
O'Conner, J.P., 60
O'Connor, J.P., 61
O'Connor, K.C., 102
Oda, S., 104, 107
Odorico, J.S., 82

Oetgen, M.E., 7
Ofek, O., 68–70, 72, 73
Ogasawara, A., 61
Ogata, N., 25
Ogata, S., 105
Ogawa, N., 61, 63
Ogawa, T., 63
Ogle, R.C., 107
Ogle, R.O., 107
Oh, B.C., 18
Oh, J., 18
Ohlsson, A., 119
Ohlsson, C., 26
Ohneda, O., 29
Ohnishi, H., 120, 122
Ohshima, H., 120, 122
Ohtani-Fujita, N., 20
Ohtsuki, C., 105
Ohtsuki, T., 75
Okada, K., 108
Okada, S., 29
Okamoto, R., 16, 17
Okamura, R.M., 21
O'Kane, S., 56
Okazaki, Y., 23
O'Keefe, J.R., 20
O'Keefe, R.J., 19, 20, 23, 26, 27, 88
Okubo, Y., 100
Okuno, M., 105
Olate, J., 18
Olsen, B.R., 16, 17
Olshanski, A., 85, 87
Olson, E.N., 18, 20
Ong, J.L., 120
Ongpipattanakul, B., 99, 104, 106
Oosterwegel, M., 21
Oreffo, R.O., 84
Orlando, P., 69
Ornelas, S.S., 62
Ornitz, D.M., 20, 26
Ornoy, A., 44
Orsini, E., 120
Orsini, G., 121
Orth, M.W., 23, 27
Osborne, J.A., 108
Ostertag, A., 75
O'Sullivan, R.J., 25, 26
Otani, T., 26
Ottani, V., 120, 122
Ott, J., 75
Otto, F., 16, 17
Oudshoorn, M.H., 107
Oukka, M., 18

Ouyang, H.J., 19
Overgaard, S., 99, 104, 106
Owen, M., 98
Owen, M.J., 16, 17, 19
Owens, M.R., 120
Owen, T.A., 16, 21
Oxlund, H., 52
Oxlun, H., 100
Oyajobi, B.O., 18
Ozawa, H., 25
Ozawa, S., 63

P
Pacifici, M., 26
Pacini, S., 53
Pajulo, O., 26
Palumbo, M., 83
Panikashvili, D., 69
Pankey, S.C., 107
Pan, W., 12
Papadopoulou, E., 56
Papaeliou, A., 56
Papagelopoulos, P.J., 62
Papalois, A., 56
Papkoff, J., 22
Paredes, R., 18
Parfitt, A.M., 121
Parhami, F., 18
Paris, M., 19
Park, H.T., 18, 105
Park, J.B., 122
Park, J.Y., 120, 122
Park, S.Y., 18
Park, Y.G., 61
Park, Y.S., 122
Park, Y.Y., 18
Parslow, T.G., 21
Parsons, J.R., 60–62
Partington, G.A., 61
Partridge, N.C., 19, 102
Paschalis, E.P., 121
Patel, M.S., 21
Pathi, S., 1, 5
Patil, S., 56
Patricelli, M.P., 69
Patt, H.M., 52
Pattison, W., 29
Pavolini, B., 1, 2, 5
Paznekas, W.A., 20
Peel, S.A.F., 121
Peet, N., 30
Peled, M., 106

Pelinkovic, D., 85, 87, 89
Pelled, G., 81–92
Pelletier, N., 18
Pelli, G., 68
Peng, H., 83, 85–87, 89
Pepato, M.T., 63
Peretti, G.M., 1, 5
Perrin-Schmitt, F., 20
Perry, M.J., 26
Pertwee, R.G., 68
Peruzzo, D., 75
Peterson, B., 85, 86
Petite, H., 100, 105
Petitet, F., 68, 71
Petrakova, K.V., 103
Petrini, M., 53
Petrosino, S., 69
Petty, E.M., 23
Pfeiffer, F., 120
Phan, D.H., 107
Phan, T.T., 104
Philbrick, W.M., 21, 22
Philipps, A.F., 25
Philipps, R., 119
Phillip, M., 23, 25
Phillips, B.W., 86
Phillips, C.L., 89
Phimphilai, M., 19
Phinney, D.G., 102
Piatetzky, S. II., 103
Piattelli, A., 121
Piattelli, M., 121
Piccari, G., 120
Pietrobon, R., 60
Pikula, S., 43, 44
Pilliar, R.M., 120
Pinzur, M.S., 62
Piomelli, D., 68, 69
Piras, F., 53
Pittenger, M.F., 82, 103
Pittman, D.D., 84, 85, 87–89
Plenk, H. Jr., 21
Plotkin, L.I., 18, 19
Pockwinse, S.M., 16, 17
Pogue, R., 26, 27
Polak, J.M., 108
Pollack, S.R., 106
Pomajzl, C., 18
Ponder, S.W., 25, 27
Poon, R., 6
Porte, D., 19
Poser, J.W., 100
Potier, E., 91
Power, J.B., 91

Powers, J.C., 60, 61
Pratap, J., 20
Prats, A.C., 53
Prats, H., 53
Prince, C.W., 63
Pritchard, J.J., 121
Probst, A., 121
Prockop, D.J., 82, 83, 102
Protivinsky, J., 120
Provot, S., 25–27
Pruchnic, R., 82, 85, 87, 89
Puleo, D.A., 121
Pulumati, M.R., 19
Puolakkainen, P.A., 107
Puukka, P., 60
Puzas, J.E., 88

Q
Qiang, Y.W., 22
Qian, Y.X., 30
Qiao, M., 18
Qi, H., 12
Quaranta, M., 120
Quarto, R., 98, 111
Quartuccio, H.A., 53
Quinn, C., 102
Quo, R.G., 21

R
Raby, N., 56
Rachmiel, A., 102, 107
Radisson, J., 44
Radomsky, M.L., 100
Rahan, S.S., 63
Rahemtulla, F., 63
Ralston, S.H., 69
Ramakrishna, S., 104
Ramirez, V., 44
Randle, W.L., 108
Rao, A., 20
Raspanti, M., 122
Rawadi, G., 22
Raye, J.R., 25
Rechenberg, B., 7
Reddi, A.H., 6, 101
Reddleman, K., 62
Reeve, J., 30
Regev, E., 12, 15, 54, 83, 85, 89
Rehnelt, J., 69
Reich, A., 107
Reilly, G.C., 30
Reinhardt, R.L., 82, 86

Reiser, J., 89
Renier, D., 20
Renshaw-Gegg, L., 29
Rethman, M.P., 83
Reyes, C.D., 120
Reyes, M., 86
Ricalton, N.S., 107
Richards, G.E., 25, 27
Richardson, J.A., 18
Richter, E.J., 120
Ricks, D.M., 89
Ricordi, C., 98
Ridge, S.A., 68
Riedel, G.E., 83
Riess, J.G., 91
Rifas, L., 102
Riggs, B.L., 83
Rigley, T., 107
Riminucci, M., 98, 99, 110
Rinaldi-Carmona, M., 68
Ritter, M.A., 62
Robbins, P., 89
Roberson, P.K., 18, 19
Roberts, A.B., 101
Roberts, E., 121
Robertson, J.A., 86
Roberts, W.E., 121
Robey, P.G., 85, 91, 98, 99, 101–103, 110
Robinson, D., 54
Robrecht, D.T., 23
Roche, N.S., 101
Rockler, B., 119
Rodan, G.A., 53, 105
Rodriguez-Avial, M., 56
Roman, A.A., 12, 13
Romano, G., 102, 108
Roman-Roman, S., 22
Ron, E., 83, 104, 106
Rönnemaa, T., 60
Rooman, R., 26
Roos, B.A., 98
Rosa, B.T., 75
Rosenblatt, M., 52
Rosen, G., 120
Rosengren, A., 121
Rosenkrantz, T.S., 25
Rosen, V., 53, 83, 100
Rosewell, I.R., 16, 17
Rosier, R.N., 88
Rosini, S., 53
Rosser, J., 121
Ross, F.P., 22, 31
Rossi, F., 69
Rossini, G., 56

Ross, R.A., 68
Roth, A.H., 26
Roussigne, M., 53
Rowe, D.W., 89
Rowe, G.C., 21, 22
Roy, S., 120
Rubin, J., 29
Rubinstein, J., 26
Rudikoff, S., 22
Rueda, C.L., 63
Ruggeri, A., 120, 122
Rupp, F., 120
Ryan, A.M., 86
Ryoo, H.M., 18, 20

S
Sabatakos, G., 21
Sadovsky, Y., 87
Sagun, R. Jr., 122
Sainson, R.C., 91
Saito, A., 105
Saito, M., 98
Sakakibara, Y., 105, 106
Sakata, T., 27
Salim, A., 91
Salisbury, K., 12, 15, 54
Saltman, L.H., 69, 72
Sampath, T.K., 100
Samuni, Y., 63
Sanchez, C., 18
Sandberg, M.M., 101
Sandborn, P.M., 120
Sander, S., 29
Sannomiya, P., 63
Sarosi, I., 30
Sasaki, A., 26
Sasaki, K., 16, 17
Sasaki, T., 21
Sassone-Corsi, P., 19
Sato, A., 121
Sato, M., 16, 17
Satomura, K., 91
Sauberlich, S., 120
Savendahl, L., 26
Sawase, T., 120
Scaf, G., 63
Scarano, A., 121
Schacht, E., 105, 107, 108
Schacht, E.H., 103
Schaefer, D., 98, 107
Schatz, A.R., 68
Schaub, R.G., 104, 106
Scheideler, L., 120

Schellander, K., 21
Scherman, D., 91
Schiller, P.C., 98
Schilling, J., 22
Schilling, T., 52, 53
Schilz, A., 89
Schindeler, A., 60
Schinke, T., 19
Schipani, E., 25–27
Schmid, C., 25, 26
Schmitz, J.P., 102, 109
Schneider, G., 120
Schneider, R.A., 1, 2, 5
Schorpp-Kistner, M., 19
Schrock, M., 20
Schroeder, A., 119
Schroeder, T.M., 16–19
Schumacker, B., 100
Schurman, L., 63
Schwartz, A.V., 60
Schwartz, Z., 25, 43, 44, 120–122
Schwarz, E.M., 19, 88
Schweitzer, P., 69
Scott, C.T., 86
Scully, S., 30
Scutt, A., 69
Secreto, F., 22
Sedlinsky, C., 63
Seedor, J.G., 53
Seeman, E., 102
Segev, E., 21
Segre, G.V., 25, 27
Seidel, J., 98, 107
Sela, J.J., 1–7, 11–32, 43–46, 52, 54, 63
Sela, M.N., 120
Selby, P.B., 16, 17
Selvamurugan, N., 19
Semba, S., 25
Senaldi, G., 30
Sennerby, L., 122
Seo, J., 19, 120
Service, R.F., 98, 105, 107
Setton, A., 43, 44
Shaaban, A.F., 82, 84
Shaftan, G.W., 60, 61
Shalabi, M.M., 119
Shalev, D.E., 69
Shalhoub, V., 16, 21, 30, 102
Shapira, L., 122
Shapiro, F., 1, 2, 5
Shapiro, I.M., 120
Shaughnessy, J.D., 22
Shea, M., 85, 104, 106, 107, 119

Shelton, J.M., 18
Sheng, M.H., 83
Shen, R., 20
Shen, V., 88
Shen, X., 121
Sherris, D.A., 106
Sheweita, S.A., 61
Sheyn, D., 92
Shibata, Y., 120
Shiga, A., 121
Shikinami, Y., 98, 105
Shiloah, S., 68
Shimada, M., 104
Shimamoto, G., 29
Shimizu, A., 86
Shimizu, E., 19
Shimizu, Y., 16, 17
Shi, M.J., 20
Shimoaka, T., 25
Shimokata, H., 75
Shimoya, K., 75
Shirakura, M., 120, 122
Shire, D., 68
Shi, Y., 21
Shoichet, M.S., 98, 106
Shteyer, A., 12, 15, 52–54
Siddiqui, A.A., 119
Sidhu, S.P., 52, 53
Sierra, J., 18
Siggelkow, H., 63
Sikavitsas, V.I., 105
Silkman, L., 61, 62
Simeonidou, C., 69
Simmons, P.J., 102
Simonet, W.S., 29, 30
Simon, G.M., 52, 53, 69
Simon, J., 102
Sims, N.A., 21
Sinal, C.J., 12, 13
Sinha, K., 19
Siniscalco, D., 69
Siqueira, J.T., 63
Sjodin, A., 68
Skerry, T.M., 30
Skillington, J., 85, 86
Skoglund, B., 56
Sleilati, G., 63
Sloan, A.J., 86
Smink, J.J., 26
Smit, A., 63
Smith, E.R., 21, 25, 27, 53
Smith, K., 56
Smith, P.A., 72, 73, 89

Smock, S.L., 21
Snyder, B., 7
Soballe, K., 99, 100, 104, 106
Sodek, J., 102, 103
Soegiarto, D.W., 25
Solheim, E., 4
Song, K.H., 61
Sonis, S.T., 106
Sonnabend, D.H., 105
Sonntag, W.E., 100
Sophocleous, A., 69
Sosic, D., 20
Soskolne, W.A., 122
Sotiropoulou, D., 120
Spelsberg, T.C., 22, 83
Spiegel, H.U., 121
Spiegelman, B.M., 15, 16
Spiekermann, H., 120
Spindler, K.P., 56
Spinella, A., 102, 108
Spires, W.P., 120
Spiro, R.C., 100
Sporn, M.B., 101
Spter, D., 25, 26
Srouji, S., 97–111
Stamatopoulos, G., 56
Stamn, T., 120
Stamp, G.W., 16, 17
Stanfield, M., 100
Starbuck, M., 21
Stark, A., 120
Staub, C., 68
Stavnezer, J., 20
Steffens, S., 68
Steger, R.W., 100
Steinberg, D., 120
Steinemann, S.G., 119
Steiner, T., 25, 26
Stein, G.S., 16–18, 20–23, 53, 69, 72, 102, 103
Stein, H., 43
Steinhardt, Y., 83, 85, 89
Stein, J.L., 16–18, 20–23
Stein, M., 43, 44
Stella, N., 69
Stemmler, M.P., 21
Stevens, D.G., 23
Stevens, H.Y., 30
Stevenson, L.A., 68
Stevenson, S., 83, 87
Stifani, S., 18
Stoetzel, C., 20
Stover, M.L., 89, 90
Strates, B.S., 100

Stratmann, U., 120
Strnad, J., 120
Strzelecka-Kiliszek, A., 43
Stubbs, D., 105
Stunkle, E., 60
Suetsugu, T., 120, 121
Sugars, R.V., 86
Suger, G., 102
Sugimoto, T., 61, 63
Sugiyama, O., 89
Suh, J.H., 18
Suh, K.T., 18
Sullivan, J., 29, 30
Sumanasinghe, R.D., 108
Sun, Y.Q., 53
Suplita, R.L., 68
Suss-Tobi, E., 98, 106, 108
Suttamanatwong, S., 22
Suva, L.J., 53
Su, X., 120
Suzuki, Y., 105
Swain, L.D., 44
Swartz, B.A., 119
Sylvia, V.L., 25, 121, 122
Sypitkowski, C., 121
Sztynda, T., 32

T
Tabata, Y., 100, 103, 105–107
Tabin, C.J., 1, 5, 25
Taddei, P., 122
Taguchi, N., 120
Taguchi, Y., 120, 122
Takagi, K., 29
Takahashi, K., 104, 107
Takaoka, K., 20
Takatsuka, S., 104
Takayanagi, H., 19, 20, 28
Takazakura, D., 104
Takeda, S., 19
Takeichi, T., 63
Takeshita, F., 120, 121
Taketomi, T., 26
Taketo, M.M., 21
Takita, H., 100
Tamai, K., 20
Tamamura, Y., 26
Tamasi, J.A., 19
Tam, J., 21, 68–70
Tamura, J., 98, 105
Tamura, M., 100, 106, 107
Tanaka, T., 120, 121

Tanaka, Y., 120
Tang, E., 21
Tangl, S., 122
Tang, Q.O., 56
Tan, H.L., 29, 30
Tanihara, M., 105
Tank, A., 21
Tapscott, S.J., 15, 16
Tarpley, J., 29
Tartakovsky, A., 53
Tashiro, H., 23
Tassinari, M., 102
Tatebe, M., 108
Tavaria, M., 32
Tavassoli, M., 52
Tawil, G., 63
Tchilibon, S., 68
Teitelbaum, S.L., 22, 31
Teixeira-Clerc, F., 68
Tellis, I., 32
Telser, J., 61
Temenoff, J.S., 105
Tenenhouse, A., 75
Tepper, G., 122
Terauchi, Y., 25
Terek, R.M., 60
Termine, J.D., 101
Testi, C., 53
Testi, R., 53
Teurich, S., 19
Thams, U., 122
Thirlwell, H., 21
Thomas, K.A., 122
Thomas, T., 83
Thompson, A.Y., 100
Thompson, B.M., 106
Thompson, D.D., 53
Thomsen, P., 119, 121
Thomson, J.A., 82
Thornell, A.P., 16, 17
Thouverey, C., 43, 44
Thrailkill, K.M., 60
Timmerman, J., 21
Timms, E., 30
Tinti, A., 122
Tintut, Y., 18
Tio, R., 63
Tokuzawa, Y., 23
Toma, C.D., 120
Tominaga, H., 19
Tong, A., 107
Tontonoz, P., 15, 16
Torricelli, P., 120

Toung, J.S., 107
Touriol, C., 53
Townes, T.M., 19
Toworfe, G.K., 120
Trail, G., 29
Tran, G.T., 56
Trantolo, D.J., 106
Trasciatti, S., 53
Tremblay, J.P., 91
Trembovler, V., 69
Triffitt, J.T., 84, 106
Trindade-Suedam, I.K., 63
Trire, A., 120
Troen, T., 30
Troiano, N.W., 7
Trombi, L., 53
Tsai, J.A., 120
Tsatsas, D., 61
Tsialogiannis, E., 56
Tsiridis, E., 3, 56
Tuckermann, J., 19
Tunes, R., 75
Tuominen, J.T., 60
Turek, T., 104, 106
Turgeman, G., 82–90
Turner, J.D., 120
Tyndall, W.A., 61
Tyson, D.R., 19

U
Uchiyama, T., 52
Ueda, M., 108
Ueki, K., 104
Ueta, C., 20
Ulrich, P., 63
Unger, C., 86
Unger, R., 103, 105, 107, 108
Upadhyay, N., 3
Urist, M.R., 83, 99, 100
Urry, Z.L., 61
Usas, A., 83, 85–87

V
Väänänen, H.K., 30, 32
Vaaraniemi, J., 32
Vaessen, B., 86
Vail, T.P., 60
Valdes, M., 83
Valentin-Opran, A., 83
Valko, M., 61
Valverde, O., 68, 71

van Buul-Offers, S.C., 26
van de Wetering, M., 21
Van, G., 29
van Geemen, D., 107
van Genderen, C., 21
Van Hoorebeke, L., 103, 107
Van Nhieu, J.T., 68
van Nostrum, C.F., 107
van Roy, F., 21
Van Sickle, D., 105
Van 't Hof, R.J., 68, 69
Van Vlierberghe, S., 103, 107
van Wijnen, A.J., 16–18, 20–23
Varady, P., 91
Varga, K., 69
Vargervik, K., 7, 106
Vayssiere, B., 22
Vega, R.B., 18
Vehof, J.W., 100
Veillard, N.R., 68
Veillette, C.J.H., 4
Velazquez, O.C., 82
Verbout, A.J., 104, 105
Vercaigne, S., 122
Verettas, D., 56
Verfaillie, C.M., 12, 86
Vermonden, T., 107
Vernochet, C., 86
Vetter, U., 25
Vidson, M., 53
Viens, M.A., 62
Viggeswarapu, M., 91
Vigorita, V.J., 52, 53
Villagra, A., 18
Villanueva, A.R., 121
Vinci, R.J., 23
Virdi, A.S., 84
Vleminckx, K., 21
Vlierberghe, S.V., 105, 108
Vocke, A.K., 121
Vogel, J.J., 43
Vogel, Z., 69
Voigt, K.H., 25
Volek-Smith, H., 83
Volinia, S., 23
von Ebner, V., 121
von Kries, J.P., 21
von Rosenheim, R., 121
Vora, S., 52
Vortkamp, A., 1, 5, 25
Vunjak-Novakovic, G., 7, 98, 107
Vuorio, E.I., 101
Vu, T.H., 86

W
Wagner, E.F., 21
Wagner, J.A., 69
Wakioka, T., 26
Wakisaka, S., 26
Wallrichs, S.L., 62
Walsh, W.R., 105
Walther, D., 75
Wang, C.K., 90
Wang, C.Y., 21
Wang, D.A., 107
Wang, E.A., 53, 83, 100
Wang, J.C., 86
Wang, L., 69, 120
Wang, Q., 19, 20
Wang, X., 22
Wang, Y.J., 20, 27
Wang, Z.Q., 21
Warman, J., 52, 53
Warshawsky, H., 120, 121
Wasan, A., 60
Wassermann, K., 87
Watazu, A., 121
Watzek, G., 122
Weber, H., 120
Wedlich, D., 21
Weinberg, H., 44
Weiner, R., 119
Wein, M.N., 18
Weinstein, R.S., 18, 19
Wei, Q., 6
Weise, M., 23
Weissman, I.L., 103
Weis, W.I., 21
Wei, X., 20
Weizmann, S., 107
Welsh, D.A., 89
Wendel, M., 86
Wennebrg, A., 122
Wennerberg, A., 122
Wenzel, A., 63
Werb, Z., 86
Wergedal, J.E., 83, 89
Westendorf, J.J., 12, 15–19, 21, 22
Whalen, J., 82, 85, 87, 89
Wheeler, S.L., 122
Whetstone, H.C., 6
White, A.A., 119
White, D.W., 52
Whitters, M.J., 100
Whyt, M.P., 75
Wieland, M., 120
Wientroub, S., 102

Wiesman, H.P., 120
Wiesmann, H.P., 120
Williams, C.G., 107
Williams, G., 69
Williamson, E.M., 69
Williams, S.M., 12
Willoughby, K.A., 69
Winchester, S.K., 19
Winnard, R.G., 120
Wisby, A., 43
Wise, D.L., 106
Wittenberg, R.H., 119
Witt, O., 53
Wittrant, Y., 61
Wobus, A.M., 86
Wolf, E., 60
Wolf, G., 63
Wolf, S., 102
Wolke, J.G.C., 119, 122
Wooden, S., 29
Woodgett, J., 21
Woodruff, K., 61, 88
Woo, K.M., 120
Wozney, J.M., 20, 53, 83, 100
Wray, J.B., 60
Wright, K.L., 21, 69, 72, 73
Wright, V., 83, 86, 87
Wronski, T.J., 100
Wu, G.J., 61
Wu, H., 20
Wuisman, P.I., 86
Wukich, D.K., 60
Wu, L., 83, 87
Wu, M., 21, 22
Wuthier, R.E., 43
Wutz, A., 21

X
Xiao, G., 19, 106
Xia, W., 91
Xie, R.L., 22
Xing, L., 20
Xu, F., 83, 87
Xu, J., 26
Xu, X., 86

Y
Yadav, V., 19
Yagi, H., 16, 17
Yagi, K., 23
Yamada, K., 106, 107
Yamada, Y., 26, 75

Yamaguchi, A., 16, 17, 83
Yamaguchi, T., 61, 63
Yamamoto, E., 104
Yamamoto, M., 61, 63, 100, 105–107
Yamamoto, T., 56
Yamashita, H., 86
Yamauchi, M., 61, 63
Yamazaki, M., 3, 61
Yang, D., 25
Yang, F., 107
Yang, I.H., 62
Yang, J.W., 102
Yang, X.J., 18–20, 86
Yang, Y., 25, 120
Yano, K., 26
Yano, S., 61, 63
Yanovski, J.A., 26
Yao, W., 100
Yaszemski, M.J., 98
Yau, T.M., 91
Yayon, A., 107
Yazulla, S., 68
Yeo, H., 18, 20
Yi, K.Y., 122
Yocum, S.A., 21
Yodoi, J., 61
Yoon, S.T., 83
Yoshiba, K., 20
Yoshida, M., 18
Yoshihara, Y., 105
Yoshiki, S., 16, 17
Yoshimura, A., 26
Yoshizawa, T., 19
Younan, R., 63
Young, B.H., 85
Young, D.W., 16, 17
Young, M.F., 101
Yudoh, K., 88
Yu, K., 20
Yu, S., 19
Yu, Y.M., 26

Z
Zabel, B.U., 16, 17
Zaidi, S.K., 16–18, 20
Zaleske, D.J., 1, 5
Zalzal, S., 120
Zambonin, C.G., 106
Zambonin, G., 106
Zarb, G.A., 119
Zarro, C., 61
Zavarselk, S., 32
Zayzafoon, M., 18, 20

Zechner, W., 122
Zeebregts, C., 63
Zhang, C., 19
Zhang, J.P., 19, 22, 85, 86
Zhang, L., 44
Zhang, M., 20, 21
Zhang, P., 75
Zhang, R., 120
Zhang, S.F., 102
Zhang, X.Y., 19, 89
Zhang, Y.Z., 22, 104
Zhang, Z., 19
Zhao, M., 18
Zhao, Q., 52

Zhao, Z., 19
Zheng, H., 61
Zhou, S., 83, 84, 86, 87, 90
Zhou, X., 19
Zhuge, Y., 82
Zhu, T., 20
Ziegler, R., 52, 53
Zilberman, Y., 83, 87, 90
Zimmer, A.M., 69, 75
Ziran, B.H., 82, 85, 87, 89
Ziv, E., 63
Zou, J., 89
Zurier, R.B., 69, 72
Zussman, E., 98, 106, 108

Subject Index

A
Adipogenic-osteoblastogenic balance, 12
Allograft bone, 98
Apoptosis, 27

B
Biodegradable matrix seeding, 103–104
BMP. *See* Bone morphogenetic protein
Bone anabolic agent
    OGP
        biosynthesis, 53, 54
        bone marrow regeneration, 52
        Erk1/2-Mapkapk2-CREB signaling
            pathway, 52–53
        fracture callus, 54, 55
        fractured femora, μCT image, 54, 55
    PTH, 51–52
    statins, 54–56
    vitamin D, 56
Bone fracture
    blood clot formation, 4
    bone repair, 1–2
    bone wound healing, 6–7
    cellular activation, signaling pathways, 3–4
    chondrogenesis, 5–6
    chronic inflammatory reaction, 4–5
    critical size defect, 7
    healing process, 1
    intramembranous and endochondral
        ossification, 4–5
    long bone fractures and callus, 2, 3
    matrix mineralization, 2
    osseous regeneration, 2
    osteoblast differentiation, 6
Bone gene therapy
    and angiogenesis, 86–87

bone formation process, 81
bone marrow-derived MSCs
    autocrine and response, 83, 84
    BMP, 83
    gene delivery vehicle, 83–84
    osteoprogenitor cell-mediated gene
        therapy, 84
    regenerative benefit, 85
    stem cell-based gene therapy, 82–83
cell source, 85–86
MSCs
    genetic engineering, 89–90
    properties, 92
    stem cell-mediated gene therapy, 90–91
multi-lineage differentiation potential, 91
nonunion defects, 81
osteogenic differentiation and
        angiogenesis, 91
osteogenic growth factor, 81
PFTBA, 91–92
stem cell, 82
systemic bone disease
    osteoclastogenesis, 88
    osteogenesis imperfecta, 88–89
    osteoporosis, 87–88
    pathology, 87
Bone morphogenetic protein (BMP)
    BMP2, 19, 83
    BMP2 signaling, 20, 22
    bone marrow-derived MSCs, 83
    chondroblast, 26–27
    osteoblast differentiation, 100
Bone repair
    adipogenic-osteoblastogenic balance, 12
    bone and cartilage cells, 11, 12
    chondroblast, 23–27
    mesenchymal stem cells, 11–12

Bone repair (*cont.*)
  osteoblasts, 13, 14
  osteoclast, 27–32
  osteocytes, 13–19
  osteogenesis regulation, microRNAs,
      22–23
  signal conduction, 11
  SMAD, 20–22
Bone tissue engineering, 107–108

C
Cannabinoid
  anandamide and 2-AG, 69
  BMD *vs.* age-matched health controls, 75
  bone cell differentiation, 71–72
  CB1 and 2-AG, bone formation, 73, 74
  CB1 and CB2, 68–69
  CB2, bone remodeling, 68, 69
  CNR2 gene, osteoporosis, 73
  CNR genes and osteoporosis relation, 75
  CNR2-mutated gene, 74–75
  endocannabinoid system
      CB2, immunnohistochemical staining,
          70, 71
      DAGL, 70, 71
      NAPE-PLD and FAAH, 70–71
  mitogenic signaling, CB2, 68–70
  sympathetic CB1 activation, 73, 74
  THC, 67–68
Cannabis sativa, 67–68
Cement lines, 121
Ceramics, 104–105
Chondroblast
  apoptosis, 27
  BMPs, 26–27
  endochondral ossification, 23, 24
  FGF, 26
  growth plate cartilage, 23, 24
  hypoxia, 27
  IGFBPs, 25
  IGF-I, 25
  Ihh, 25
  intrinsic paracrine factors, 23, 25
  PTHrP, 25–26
  TGFβ, 26
  Wnt protein, 26
Chondrogenesis, 5–6

D
Diabetes mellitus
  callus formation, etiology, 60
  delayed fracture healing, 60

DM and bone metabolism, 60
  fracture, complications, 62
  histological stages, 59–60
  hyperglycosylation, 63
  insulin, anabolic effect, 60–61
  insulin therapy, 61–62
  orthopedic and dental implant, 62–63
  oxidative stress, 61
  WNT pathway, 61

E
Endocannabinoid system
  CB2, immunnohistochemical staining, 70, 71
  DAGL, 70, 71
  NAPE-PLD and FAAH, 70–71
Endochondral ossification, 4–5, 23

F
Firoblast growth factor (FGF), 6, 26
Fracture. *See* Bone fracture
Fracture callus, 54, 55, 60, 61, 100–101

G
Genetic engineering, 89–90

H
Hydroxyapatite (HA) crystal
  collagen rich matrix, 44, 45
  crystal formation, 43–44
Hypoxia, 27

I
IGF-binding proteins (IGFBPs), 25
Implants, bone reaction
  biocompatibility, 120
  cement lines, 121
  heterogeneity, 121
  hydroxyapatite coating, 122
  implant stability, 119–120
  osseointegration, 119
  osteoclast TEM images, 121
  osteoconductivity, 120
  titanium alloy (Ti) implant, 119
Indian hedgehog (Ihh), 24, 25

M
Matrix vesicle (MV) mineralization
  electron opaque MV, 44, 45

HA crystal, collagen rich matrix, 44, 45
HA crystal formation, 43–44
hydroxyapatite crystallization, 43
mineralization process, 44, 46
osteoblast, 44, 46
primary mineralization, 43
proteomic analysis, 43
vesicular life cycle, 44
Mesenchymal stem cells (MSCs)
    bone marrow-derived MSCs
        autocrine and paracrine response, 83,
            84
        BMP, 83
        gene delivery vehicle, 83–84
        osteoprogenitor cell-mediated gene
            therapy, 84
        regenerative benefit, 85
        stem cell-based gene therapy, 82–83
    genetic engineering, 89–90
    osteogenic differentiation and
        angiogenesis, 91
    properties, 92
    stem cell-mediated gene therapy, 90–91
MSCs. See Mesenchymal stem cells
MV mineralization. See Matrix vesicle
    mineralization

N
Native polymers, 105

O
OGP. See Osteogenic growth peptide
Osteoclast
    histology, 27–28
    M-CSF-RANKL system, 28, 29
    migration and targeting, 29–30
    mineral dissolution, 31
    mineralized tissue resorption, 32
    osteoclastic bone resorption, 31–32
    resorbing osteoclast, 30
    resorption product disposal, 32
    stromal cell-osteoclast interaction, 28–29
Osteocyte
    ATF4, 19
    E11/gp38 molecule, 16
    impregnation methodology, 13, 14
    mineralized matrix, electron micrograph,
        13, 15
    myogenic path, 16
    osteocytic processes, TEM, 13, 15
    osterix, 19
    Runx2, 17–18

Runx2 and HDAC interaction, 18–19
sequential marker-gene expression, 17–18
shear stress and prostaglandin
    release, 15
transcription and epigenetic co-regulators,
    16–17
Osteogenesis imperfecta, 88–89
Osteogenic growth peptide (OGP)
    biosynthesis, 53, 54
    bone marrow regeneration, 52
    Erk1/2-Mapkapk2-CREB signaling
        pathway, 52–53
    fracture callus, 54, 55
    fractured femora, μCT image, 54, 55
Osterix (Osx), 19

P
Parathyroid hormone (PTH), 51–52
PTH related protein (PTHrP), 25–26

S
Skeletal repair
    allograft bone, 98
    autogenous cancellous bone, 98
    bioreactors, 105–106
    bone defect repair and growth factors
        biomechanical properties vs. bone
            formation, 102
        bone morphogenetic protein, 99–100
        cell-scaffold construct, 99
        fracture healing, 100–101
        skeletal progenitor cell, 100, 101
        TGF-β + IGF-1, 101–102
    bone marrow stem cells, 102–103
    bone marrow stem cells-based transplants,
        97–98
    bone tissue engineering,
        107–108
    cell-scaffold construct, 98–99
    3D scaffold, 97
    fracture healing, 98
    osteoprogenitor cell, 97
    scaffold biodegradation, 106–107
    scaffolds and biomaterials
        biodegradable matrix
            seeding, 103–104
        ceramics, 104–105
        composites, 105
        native polymers, 105
        synthetic polymers, 104
        types, 104
    segmental bone repair, 106

Skeletal repair (*cont.*)
   in vivo preclinical test
      bone repair, animal model, 109
      critical size defect, 109–110
      experimental model, 109–110
      MSCs-based implants, 110–111
      osteogenic differentiation stages, 111
SMAD
   AP-1, 21
   BMP/Runx2-mediated
      osteogenesis, 20
   NFATc1/calcineurin, 20
   Tcf7/Lef1 transcription
      factor, 21–22
   Twist, 20
   ZFP, 22
Statins, 54–56
Synthetic polymers, 104
Systemic bone disease
   osteoclastogenesis, 88

osteogenesis imperfecta, 88–89
osteoporosis, 87–88
pathology, 87

T
TGFβ, 26

V
Vitamin D, 56

W
Wnt pathway, 61
Wnt protein, 26

Z
Zinc finger proteins (ZFP), 22